The Bond Effect

Natural Eating

Eating in harmony with our genetic programming
Deep down you know it makes sense!

Geoff Bond

With a Foreword by
Dr. Christopher C. Brown
Director of the Sheridan Research Institute

Griffin Publishing Group
Torrance, California

Editor: Tom Pickering
Director Of Operations: Robin L. Howland
Project Manager: Bryan K. Howland
Book Design: Midnight Media
Cover Design: m2 design group/Eleanor Reagh

10 9 8 7 6 5 4 3 2 1
ISBN 1-58000-054-1

Griffin Publishing Group
2908 Oregon Court, Suite I-5
Torrance, CA 90503
Phone: (310) 381-0485
Fax: (310) 381-0499

Geoff Bond
The Bond Effect
www.thebondeffect.com

Manufactured in the United States of America

This book is not intended to replace medical advice or to be a substitute for a physician. Always seek the advice of a physician before beginning any diet program. The author and the publisher expressly disclaim responsibility for any adverse effects arising from following the diet program in this book without appropriate medical supervision.

Acknowledgements

This book is the culmination of a long journey. Many people have helped me along the way and it is my pleasure here to single out some of them for special mention. If you are one of the many meritorious contributors whom it has not been possible to cite, just know that you are, like Henry V's unsung heroes, "freshly remember'd" and that your influence lives on in this work.

First of all, thanks to Nicole my wife. She is my most ardent disciple and proselytizer. With her fervent belief in the importance to humanity of the insights contained in these pages, she has supported me through the difficult gestation process. She has appraised every word of the text with her Teutonic thoroughness. If any part remains obscure, deficient or sesquipedalian then it is not for want of her cajoling. Nicole's support, advice, criticism and encouragement have been invaluable.

An early, and surely essential, influence was that of my gritty, selfless grandmother, Anna Svehla. At her knee we learned to respect our bodies and think critically about what we put in our mouths. She pluckily challenged the purblind dietary doctrines of her day. She was decades ahead of her time and predictably, as pioneers do, had a hard time of it.

This book would not have been possible without the peculiarities of upbringing that created in me an untamed questioning, a delight in discovery and a distaste for flummery. Thank you then, to my undoctrinaire parents who allowed me to fossick on my own and who taught me the value of 'per ardua ad astra' (through hard work to the stars).

I am indebted too to the many key people, acolytes all, who, at the right moment and in their many ways, brought me to this point in the journey:
— Brent Lance, whose excitement, expert guidance and encouragement in the early days launched me into systematizing the Bond Effect for the benefit of the general public,
— Joe Schuchert, whose conviction, determination and foresight brought these insights to corporate America,
— Emmanuel Kampouris, aided by his wife Camille, whose courage, persistence and vision brought the precursor to this book, the Introductory Guide to tens of thousands of people,
— Dickson Buxton, who has generously deployed his wealth of experience to develop the presence of Natural Eating in the USA,
— Dan Wilson and Gary MacDonald who have devoted much of their spare time and sage expertise to promulgate the Natural Eating message,
— Don Harper, who had the clarity of purpose and confidence in me to expand our impact in the United Kingdom,
— Frederic Bouvet, who has worked altruistically and imaginatively to bring knowledge of the Natural Eating precepts to the populations of Continental Europe,
— Ingeborg Hoss, whose delicate drawings adorn three of these pages. Mention too for the hospitality of her atmospheric Provençale farmhouse where much of this book was written.

To all of you, and to all of those as yet unsung, my heartfelt thanks.

C o n t e n t s

F o r e w o r d

By Dr. Christopher C. Brown

The field of nutrition, as we know it, is currently undergoing remarkable scrutiny. Dogmatic theories and tenets are becoming suspect in the face of innovative research by new thinkers like Geoff Bond.

I am intrigued by recent works which call into question the presumed healthy nature of our carbohydrate-laden diet. I have read all the books; the Atkins diet, Sugar Busters, The Zone and Protein Power. Then I had the pleasure of reading a new book, Natural Eating, written by British nutritional anthropologist, Geoff Bond.

This book is a remarkable treatise; a well-researched and well thought out critique of the "modern diet". To date, it provides the most convincing and scientifically intact indictment of the high-carbohydrate diet. Rather than focusing exclusively on the issue of carbohydrates, Natural Eating deals with all aspects of nutrition, providing extensive and convincing scientific support from both the basic science and social science literature.

Over the last couple of years I have been so convinced by Geoff's work that I have applied the principles to my own diet as well as those of my patients. I can personally attest to the remarkable effects attainable. In my own case, I noted an improved sense of well-being, increased energy, weight loss and improved blood lipid profile. I have recommended the diet to a number of patients with remarkable results, especially in diabetics, overweight and hyperlipidemic individuals. I fully endorse Natural Eating and suggest and hope that it will have a significant impact on the future of nutrition as we know it.

Christopher C. Brown, M.D.

Dr. Christopher Brown, Director of the Sheridan Research Institute, is board-certified in both Internal Medicine and Infectious Diseases. He spent a number of years doing research at the National Institutes of Health. For the last seven years he has run a busy private practice in Internal Medicine.

Preface

"**Man, alone amongst the living creatures, tries to deny the laws of nature.**"

Why: do the Japanese live much longer than Americans?

Why: were our prehistoric forebears taller than we are today?

What: is it about the Greeks that they are healthier than Americans?

Why: do some people think it is normal to have: bad digestion, constipation, arthritis, cellulite, heart disease, obesity, osteoporosis?

Think about this:

When you go to the zoo, there are signs:

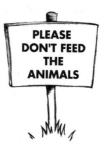

The zookeepers know that the animals have to be fed with foods that are appropriate to their species!

> **This book is about defining and practicing the feeding patterns appropriate to our species.**

Introduction

Important Concepts

The basic premise of Natural Eating is eating in a way which is in harmony with the way our bodies have been designed. It is like finding the right quality of gas to put into your car, only much more complex!

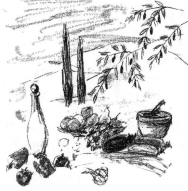

The conclusions we arrive at have some daunting implications. Most of us need to restructure how and what we eat. The good news is that small adjustments can make a big difference! How many of us suffer from acid stomach, flatulence or constipation? There are ready and rapid solutions to these conditions.

By making other adjustments, you can achieve rapid weight loss, while improving your health and life chances. Additionally, you can increase your resistance to cancer, obesity, diabetes, arthritis, osteoporosis, cardiovascular problems and other degenerative diseases.

---◆---

Natural Eating is about realizing your full potential for good health and prolonging youth into old age.

---◆---

The message is work your way through this book and decide how much restructuring you can and want to live with. This process will tell what changes to make as a priority and what eating pleasures you can safely keep. Because it will still be possible to eat well but *differently*. It will be possible to pick one habit, modify it, get the new habit established and move on to the next. Take it at your own pace and stop when you like.

---◆---

This book presents the ideal to aim at.

How much you do or how far you go is up to you.

---◆---

Who Can Benefit From Natural Eating?

Everybody

If you are a human being, you qualify to enjoy the benefits of Natural Eating. Healthy or sick, slim or overweight, old or young, male or female, you will find within these pages the eating strategies to maximize your health and longevity.

- Starting young is even better
- Think of youngsters who can benefit
- It is never too late to start

The Natural Eating precepts are solidly grounded in intellectual rigor and scientific discovery. There is no place here for mysticism, wishful thinking or self-delusion. There is a wind of change blowing through the nutritional establishment. It is gradually being recognized that the only way to understand our ideal feeding pattern is to go back to our origins. Our bodies are designed to work best with a particular kind of fuel and we have lost the specification. This book is abut the rediscovery of that specification.

We all feel bombarded by messages, most of them conflicting, about what and how we should be eating. Many of the messages are put out by commercial interests who deliberately make you anxious to buy their products. Using the powerful tools provided by the Natural Eating vantage point, you can bring clarity to the confusion and clarity to the conflicting messages jostling for your attention.

◆

The Natural Eating precepts bring clarity to the multitude of conflicting messages jostling for our attention

◆

The broad principles in this book apply to everybody, though certain groups may have particular concerns.

The Sick And Overweight

Chapter Eight, The Food/Disease Connection, covers a broad range of diseases aggravated by dietary errors, including obesity, and prioritizes the changes to be made.

Special Age-groups

There are phases in life when special attention is paid to health matters. Chapter Six, The Method, explains how Natural Eating applies to babies and toddlers, children and adolescents, pregnant and nursing women, thirty-somethings, menopausal women, the elderly.

Special Dietary Practices

This book focuses purely on the eating patterns for which humans are naturally adapted. Nevertheless, there are other dimensions to our eating decisions:

For example, there can be religious prescriptions, such as the avoidance of pork, and there can be ethical reasons.

Ethical reasons are those such as wanting to be eco-friendly or avoiding cruelty to animals. Other reasons are wanting to avoid food contaminants such as hormones and pesticides and bio-engineered foods like G.M.O's (genetically modified organisms).

Such people can overlay these requirements onto the Natural Eating Pattern. The composite pattern that is right for them will emerge. Those following religious or ethical eating patterns will find within these pages the map to optimum health.

Although a strong case can be made for a meatless eating pattern in today's world, this is not a book that promotes the cause of vegetarianism. Meatless eating is more than just leaving meat out of the diet. It means severely curtailing other food groups too and making significant adjustments to the remaining components of the food intake.

For this reason, a segment on vegetarian diet is found in Chapter Six.

C h a p t e r   O n e

Connecting the Dots

As a small boy in war-torn Britain, I lived with my grandparents. My grandmother was a special person. A vegetarian with a mission. She strongly believed in eating lots of raw fruit and vegetables. Even in wartime Britain, sliced raw carrots, celery sticks and cucumbers were constantly on the table. If I felt hungry, I only had to fill up as I ran past the bowl of raw salads.

War over, father back from the Indian front and all back in the family home, the same eating patterns were maintained. Growing up, I would be known as "baby face" due to my clear complexion and cheeks glowing with good health. Strong, well muscled and stocky, I was never off sick. But like any eight year old I was a ripe subject for any idea, good or bad, that wanted to take up residence in my mind.

———— ◆ ————

Ideas, good or bad, readily take up residence in a youngster's mind.

———— ◆ ————

At school I read glossy brochures, produced by the Milk Marketing Board extolling the calcium-bearing virtues of dairy products. "Milk and cheese are vital for a growing child - they help build bones!"

It was then that my interest in nutrition began.

But there was a problem. Our family abstained from dairy products. To drink milk was, to me, as bizarre and unpleasant as taking cod-liver oil! In fact, when I was forced to drink the school milk[1], it made me throw up. At school I was treated as an ungrateful oddball.

Those well-meaning teachers were determined that I shouldn't suffer a calcium deficiency. "Drink up your milk," they said. "It's good for you!"

But having a small kid throw up over you isn't much fun, even for a hardened infant teacher. After a short battle, I remained gloriously milk-free, even at school.

Yet here I was, an eight year old "not getting his calcium because he doesn't drink milk." My father brought down from the bookshelf a copy

---

1 In the newly installed welfare state, all children not only had the right, but the duty, to consume the one third imperial pint of milk per day that was provided free of charge to schools.

of the MAFF[2] Manual of Nutrition. This was (and still is) a guide to the current 'orthodox' wisdom on eating for good health.

From this book I learned that the British diet was considered by the 'authorities' to be deficient in calcium. To remedy this, the government had ordained that powdered chalk should be added to the white flour used for making bread.

I drew the obvious conclusion – eat more white bread - and if possible add yet more chalk to it!

Reassurance was found in the MAFF food composition tables. Sardines, with their bones, contained calcium. My parents were less strict than my grandmother, and the first compromise was made. Fish entered my diet, and we had sardines on toast for tea several times a week.

I was only eight years old, and I had not fully developed the skepticism needed to properly interpret this information. Even at that tender age, I was uneasy at the assumption that, by eating a sardine's bones, they would somehow find their way into my bones.

This was also the first example too of a common phenomenon. In wanting to do better, I was meddling in matters I only half understood. I had rejected the wholewheat bread, the staple of my earlier years for the nutritionally inferior (but calcium 'enriched') white bread.

Since World War II, governments everywhere have been ordaining that more and more nutrients be added to the staple foods of their peoples. It was only decades later that I started to question this practice. Why is the average diet deficient in so many minerals and vitamins? Why is it that staples like bread, flour, and breakfast cereals have to be 'enriched'?

Around the same time, I was getting awkward questions from schoolfriends' parents about protein. "What did we do for protein?" It bothered me that slogans were urging us to eat lamb chops "for the protein". The MAFF food tables reassured me. Protein is present in nearly all vegetation, particularly the omnipresent baked beans of the post war diet.

It was much later that I discovered that this simplistic approach to nutrition by itself is not enough. Just because this or that molecule can be detected by a laboratory test doesn't mean that the body is going to make use of it. Furthermore, there are many molecules essential to health, which haven't even been identified yet. Indeed, one of the extraordinary gaps in human knowledge, is our ignorance about what exactly is in food, how our bodies absorb food and the uses our body makes of it.

But we are getting ahead of the story.

I became fascinated with body and food chemistry. I had my own

2 Ministry of Agriculture, Fisheries and Food.

laboratory in the tool shed and regularly came top of the class. I was well on my way to becoming a mechanistic food scientist dreaming of the day when we could get all our nutrients from a couple of tablets.

My doubts started during my first university work-placement with a large brewery company. I worked in the laboratory, the sole function of which was to discover ever cheaper ingredients to replace the hops and malt from which beer is traditionally made. I was aghast at the 'progress' that had been made.

This nationally drunk beer was nothing more than fermented sugar-water with a variety of flavourings and colourings. But even that was not cheap enough for the brewer. There was still a colouring that was unacceptably expensive – caramel. It was used to give the fermented sugar-water a dark 'beer' colour. Our mission was to find a cheaper substitute for the expensive substitute!

Deservedly, this beer finally lost all credibility with the drinking public. Sales went flat and it was withdrawn from the market. Nevertheless, in my wildest dreams I never imagined that the same process might also be happening to fundamentally important staple foods like bread.

Another university work-placement found me in Zaragoza, Spain, a large regional town. In the early sixties, Spain was still a poor country, frozen in a pre-civil war, General Franco, time-warp.

I was billeted with a Spanish family. Wanting to please me they asked what I liked for breakfast. I had not liked the pungent oil that came with the hard Spanish bread, so I asked if they had any butter.

They looked at each other in puzzlement. I checked with the English-Spanish dictionary to make sure of the word and showed it to them. They were even more puzzled, so they looked up the word in a Spanish language dictionary. There they found the definition of "butter."

These Spaniards, a European people who had colonized large parts of the world, a people who had battled England down the centuries, *had hardly heard of butter!*

This was my first encounter with the notion that dairy products are regarded by most peoples of the world as an exotic and bizarre foodstuff.

It was at about this same time that many West Indians migrated to Britain. A circular went out to the schools advising "don't insist that these newcomers drink the school milk; many of them are intolerant of it." Official recognition at last! But what about the rest of us?

It was a question to be answered later, but fortune took a turn. I was much inspired by the stories of the great explorations. Of "taming the great forces of nature for the use and purpose of man..[3]" I determined to study

3 Motto of the Institution of Civil Engineers.

the hard sciences and develop the skills to contribute to underdeveloped parts of the world.

I had visions of climbing mountain ranges with a theodolite, laying down the first routes of railway lines and canals. I was imbued with the spirit of the pioneering types who had opened up obscure parts in remote continents. Like Dr. Livingstone, I would live among the local population, live as they did, speak their language.

When I had finished those professional qualifications, I did indeed bring water supply to remote villages, and hack out the lines of new roads through the bush – West Africa, North Africa and the Middle East.

All the while my interests in the peoples, languages and cultures were dominant. I wanted to know their histories, their ancient migrations, their cultural identities. Above all, I was looking for some common nutritional theme.

I continued my travels: Asia, Polynesia, Australasia. My lifelong assumptions about dietary eating patterns came under pressure. Everywhere I went, people ate a wide variety of foodstuffs. Some peoples seemed to do better than others. But universally, when an early culture adopted Western eating habits, their health deteriorated and their life-span shortened. How could this be? Is it that different peoples are adapted to different eating patterns?

There had only been a couple of thousand generations since the initial Homo sapiens dispersal out of Africa 50,000 years ago. Enough certainly for superficial racial differences to come about, but little more than that. Is the Western diet just as bad, then, for Westerners?

On one occasion I was invited to eat with a Berber tribal chieftain in the Atlas mountains of Morocco. Being a special occasion, it was to be a great feast. We were to eat a 'mechoui' – a baked ram. Smoldering embers were put in a hollow in the earth. The whole sheep was placed on the embers and the lot covered over with earth. It was left to cook for several hours.

The roasted ram was presented, still whole, on a huge brass platter with little indentations around the rim. Each indentation served to hold a spice: cumin, pepper, saffron, pimento… There were dozens.

The chief presided and personally buried his hands into the roasted flesh and pulled out the choice parts for distribution. I was guest of honour, and watched in horror as he peeled the testicles out of their membrane and handed them to me. Me a quasi-vegetarian!

I made a valiant effort to show enthusiasm as I played at nibbling on a morsel while the chief regarded me with generous bonhomie. As soon as he averted his gaze, I slipped these choice morsels under the rim of the brass platter.

I looked around for something else to eat. There was nothing. No French fries, no rice, not even any cous-cous, much less was there any sign of green vegetables. Just the roast sheep - that was it. It was a lesson that I was to learn many times over. When some cultures eat meat, they eat it on its own. Halfway around the world, the cannibalistic Fijians used to cook and serve their grisly human meal in exactly the same way. Not a French fry in sight!

It was not until much later that I came across the physiological justification for keeping certain foodstuffs separate from others. Popular diet books were recycling the early theories of Dr. Shelton and of the even earlier Dr. Hay. They suggested that food separation is an important element in controlling indigestion, ill health and obesity.

Why hadn't I heard about food separation? I looked up my old college books on human nutrition. There, mentioned in passing, would be little nuggets: "...to be digested, starch needs an alkaline environment, protein needs an acid environment. It is as well ...[to eat] starchy foods at the end of the meal[4]."

So the notion that it is advisable to pay attention to how different types of food react with each other was acknowledged back in 1948! This diffident throwaway phrase was just the tip of the iceberg. Slowly the huge complexity of the digestive process is being uncovered, and the physiological basis for what is now known as 'the principle of proper food combining' is being established.

Meanwhile, I had been keeping up with my professional journals. Discoveries were being made on many fronts. It was found that the peoples who first developed agriculture by growing cereals in the Middle East, 10,000 years ago, must have done so under duress. Indeed they had phases of doing it and then abandoning it over a couple of centuries. Grinding the seeds to flour was found to be hard work. Their bones showed abnormal wear and tear. They lost stature, their lifespan shortened. Why did they put up with it then?

There was speculation about how they ate the flour that they made. (It would be another 3,000 years before bread was invented.) From my knowledge of the Aborigines, I knew the answer: the Aborigines, when times are really bad, will collect seeds and grind them between two stones. The resulting flour is moulded into patties and baked in the embers of a fire. The cooking is important because humans don't secrete the enzymes to digest raw flour.

4 Human Nutrition; Barasi & Mottram; Hodder & Stoughton.

I thought about this: *humans are not naturally adapted to the consumption and digestion of grains.* Does this mean that our bio-chemistry is also put under stress by these foods?

More discoveries were being made about our early ancestors in our ancient homeland on the edges of the tropical rain forest in East Africa. We understood more about the ways they must have lived and their eating patterns. I pondered the fact that it is only 2,000 generations since our ancestors left the area. Our bodies are, to all intents and purposes, the same.

What were these Pleistocene ancestors eating? Clearly they were 'browsing' the land for whatever they could find. Researches were showing that they weren't the great hunters that they were cracked up to be, so meat was not such an important part of the diet. But research was also showing that the nature of wild meat is quite different from the meat in the supermarket today.

On one of my trips back to London, I had a dental check up. It was a new dentist, a South African. After he had finished his inspection he said "You have a very healthy mouth and very strong teeth – just like an African's."

"What do you mean by that," I asked.

He answered a bit vaguely, "Africans have a saliva that has a better balance and it kills bacteria."

When I pressed him for more details he couldn't be more precise. I looked into it. Now we know that even the quality of the saliva in your mouth can be undermined by eating habits that diverge from our naturally adapted ones. But what are these naturally adapted eating patterns?

Other clues were coming out from bio-chemistry and population studies. Plainly, certain foodstuffs, ones that we in the West took for granted, were having a detrimental effect on health. An early bad guy was cholesterol. He was followed in quick succession by saturated fat. Study after study showed that the consumption of saturated fat was implicated in heart disease, cancer and even arthritis and allergies.

Study after study was also showing that people who had higher levels of fruit and vegetable intake were also the healthiest and longest lived.

I had seen that rural Africans, who ate a lot of dietary fibre, didn't suffer at all from intestinal diseases such as constipation, diverticulosis and colon cancer. These casual observations were backed up by ground-breaking scientific papers. Other studies showed that cereal fibre is less good than the 'soluble' fibre found in colored plant food. This interesting nuance, on the sorts of plant fibers to which human beings are best adapted, is dealt with in Chapter Four.

At the start of the Eighties I heard of the pioneering studies on blood sugar tolerance. The results rocked those few members of the medical community who paid attention. These studies demonstrated that extremely common foodstuffs like cereals, grains, potatoes and sugars put an enormous stress on the body's ability to control blood sugar levels. Many people's control mechanism couldn't cope, and as a result they were sick, sometimes gravely so.

Since then, a series of studies has deepened and widened our understanding of this phenomenon. Clearly, the human body was not naturally adapted to these foodstuffs. That was why Eskimos, Aborigines, Navajos, Polynesians and many others suffered from obesity and diabetes when they 'acculturated' to a high carbohydrate Western diet. And now Westerner's health was caving under the onslaught too!

Are there any other drawbacks to these foods? My mind went back to my childhood. Of eating bread because of the added calcium. Of seeing more and more minerals and vitamins required by law to 'enrich' various cereal products.

The scales fell from my eyes. These staples – wheat, bread, rice, breakfast cereals – these foodstuffs that 'everyone knew' were an essential part of the diet are nothing of the sort. They are foodstuffs that can only be made fitter for human consumption by the addition of a myriad of ever-increasing micro-nutrients!

————— ◆ —————

So-called staples are so deficient in micro-nutrients that governments require their 'enrichment'.

————— ◆ —————

Note the word "fitter". Even with government ordained additives, these staples of the Western diet are still only impoverished substitutes for the 'real thing'. But what is the real thing?

By this time, I was a high-powered executive jetting around the globe, struggling with airline meals, hotel restaurants, and a jet-lagged digestive system. I was still disgustingly healthy, but I was struggling to control 7 pounds of excess weight.

I took time out to go back into the bowels of the British Library and seek out all knowledge of human eating patterns.

In even scientific thinking, a common wisdom once rooted was difficult to dislodge – even with hard evidence. With difficulty, researchers of early hominid eating patterns were struggling to be heard about their findings. Since my formative years in the 1960s, it had been found that humans had been much more 'gatherers' than 'hunters'.

I came across Victorian explorers accounts of Eskimo eating patterns. I re-

read the 1930s scientific articles that described experiments on two arctic explorers. These hardy volunteers lived in the metabolism ward of Bellevue Hospital, New York, and ate nothing but fatty meat, some of it raw, for an entire year! Their vital signs were followed, regularly measured and at the end of the experiment relatively up-beat conclusions drawn about the impact on their health.

But all studies are not equal in value. Some are well done, some are sloppy. Some types of study are inherently more credible than others. Many studies are tainted by the prejudices of the researchers who conclude that their pet theories are confirmed in spite of the evidence to the contrary. By now I was used to reading the fine print and checking out who paid for the study. This one was sponsored by the Institute of American Meat Packers!

There, buried in the results, was the fact that these subjects were in constant negative calcium balance. Does a high meat diet equate to bone demineralization?

I revisited all my professional journals. What do we know about aboriginal and ancient Egyptian eating patterns? What was the latest from the forensic archaeologists on the nutritional status and diets of our prehistoric ancestors?

How do our digestive system, our jaws and our teeth compare with those of carnivores, granivores (cereal eaters), and lactivores[5] (unweaned babies). How do they compare to those of creatures that are built to very similar body plans like the great apes? The blueprint for building a gorilla (its DNA) is virtually identical (98%) to the blueprint for building a human being.

Bit by bit I joined up all the dots. And bit by bit the picture took shape. This was not an easy process for me. Later in this book I write about confronting your prejudices. I know what that means because I have had to confront my own. My early conditioning had me believing that human beings were natural vegetarians. But as each piece of evidence thudded into place, it was quite clear that 'animal matter' had played a modest but essential part of our naturally adapted diet. There is a lot later in this book about the nature of this animal matter and how the meat of today is nothing like it. It was small comfort for me to realize that the Western diet is harmful in part, not because we eat meat, but because it is the wrong kind. We also eat far too much of it.

Once I had come to terms with this awkward truth, I was able to stand back and view the complete image the picture of the eating pattern to which humankind is naturally adapted.

---

5 The term lactivore is applied to natural consumers of milk. Inevitably, this applies uniquely to the unweened young of a species. Once weened their bodies are just not adapted to milk as a food. Humans are the only creatures that attempt to deny this reality by continuing milk consumption (and that of other species to boot) into adulthood.

———— ◆ ————

The last piece of the jig-saw fell into place to reveal the naturally adapted eating pattern.

———— ◆ ————

Yet that was only the beginning. How did this pattern square with what other scientists were finding out about healthful eating practices? There are literally hundreds of thousands of scientific studies published in 'peer review' journals. These are (or should be) the gold standard for reporting the results of experiments with integrity, honesty and the absence of wishful thinking.

I collected and sifted through thousands of such articles. One major group is on *clinical feeding trials.* The best of such trials are 'double blind,' and, where practicable, with 'cross-over' carried out on at least several hundred people divided into two groups – a test group for the new diet, and a control group that continues to eat in its traditional way.

Sometimes these studies go on for many years at least five and preferably ten. Occasionally the results are so dramatic that the trial is finished early to enable the control group to benefit from the health insights of the test group.

Another major group concerns *epidemiological studies.* These are studies that examine whole populations and look at how their health is affected by diet and other factors.

Though human beings are basically tropical creatures, we now live in places that are not tropical, and we live on a multitude of different dietaries. Today the planet is like a huge laboratory with experiments going on in different corners. It is an ideal opportunity to statistically study how different lifestyles affect health and longevity.

Such studies are intriguing and highlight trends, although they are inherently less precise than clinical studies. One difficulty is to separate out what are known as 'confounding factors'. For example, the Japanese have a much longer life-expectancy than Americans but they smoke a lot more too! Do the Japanese possess this longevity because of, or in spite of, their smoking habit?

Today there are fancy statistical methods for filtering out these effects and clear trends can be identified.

To recapitulate, a multitude of scientific studies were examined. Some of them are better done than others. In some of them you have to read between the lines or even call up the researcher to find out what had been censored by the peer-review panel. All studies had to be regarded through the lens of healthy skepticism.

Nevertheless, when all was said and done, the sum total of these studies pointed in the same direction toward the naturally adapted eating pattern that I had identified earlier.

Wonderful!

However, there is one small problem… we live in today's world. We no longer 'browse' on the edge of a tropical rain forest, we now browse in the aisles of a supermarket. Do human instincts and lore, honed over millions of years to select the right foodstuff in the east African savannah serve us well in a fast food restaurant? Clearly not!

The second half of my challenge lay before me. How to identify and *prioritize* the food choices that today's hominid must make every day. What to make of all the novelties that have crept into the human diet for millennia? What to make of: caffeine, wine, maple syrup, pastries, processed foods, microwave meals, bologna sausage, Nutrasweet™, pizzas and thousands of other products put before us?

Back again to the bowels of the British Library, to my professional publications and to the food manufacturers. The latter are helpful, up to a point. They cheerfully tell you everything that the law obliges them to divulge, or that is to their advantage. They are very secretive about everything else. It is a scandal that they are allowed to sell, for *consumption* no less, products of which the precise content and processing are secret. It has to be the last industry where the vendor gets away with selling a pig in a poke!

Over a period of several years I sifted, sorted and categorized a wide variety of novel foodstuffs. That is to say, foodstuffs that have entered the human diet for the first time since the agricultural revolution 10,000 years ago. I have examined them to understand what, if any, drawbacks or advantages they have.

Finally, the fruits of this endeavour took shape in the development of the principles of 'Natural Eating'. It is the pattern of eating, as can be practiced in today's world, to which the human race is naturally adapted.

This philosophy has generated widespread interest and many successful followers. What does it entail? How does one practice it? What are the benefits? The purpose of the rest of this book is to answer these questions!

——————— ◆ ———————

Natural Eating is the pattern of eating that is in harmony with our genetic programming.

——————— ◆ ———————

C h a p t e r   T w o

The Rewards

"Courage to the Sticking-Place" – William Shakespeare

You will no doubt be thinking that Natural Eating demands a revolution in eating habits. And, carried to its ultimate perfection, it does. The good news however, is that it can be done by degrees, and every shift in the right direction will bring its benefits.

— ◆ —

Every shift in the right direction will bring new benefits

— ◆ —

In Chapter Ten, *The Ten Steps to Success*, the 'shifts' to take are given in priority order. That way you can start easily and work up to your level of comfort.

One of the hardest things to do is to confront our own prejudices and to swim against the tide of our own cultural traditions. Remember however, that it is your own health and well-being that is at stake. Our eating habits today are almost entirely culture specific.

— ◆ —

Our eating habits are mainly the result of cultural programming.

— ◆ —

The great Arctic explorer, Amundsen, on his expeditions to the North pole used to live on frozen raw seal the skin, the blood, the guts, everything – just like his Eskimo mentors. He was asked, "How could you do that?" Amundsen replied "People like what they are used to eating." *He had to get used to liking a different pattern of eating.*

— ◆ —

People like to eat what they are used to eating.

— ◆ —

This book is not about getting you to eat like an Eskimo – almost the opposite! It is about getting you to like eating *differently.*

The following pages are an overview of the kinds of benefit that can be expected by eating naturally – eating in accordance with our genetic programming. In Chapter Eight, *The Food/Disease Connection*, the maladies mentioned here are looked at in greater depth. This chapter is to remind you of the rewards of Natural Eating.

Weight Control

However much we delude ourselves, it is quite *unnatural* as well as *unhealthy* to be overweight. Indeed, the people who are the healthiest and live the longest, have the lowest percentages of body fat.

It is true that we are genetically programmed to eat large volumes of food, but they are the low calorie-dense ones like fruit and vegetation. Today we stuff ourselves with the wrong kinds of foods, the *high* calorie-dense ones like meat, fat and bad carbohydrates.

Returning to the eating patterns to which our bodies are designed will ensure that our bodies will return to the shape they were intended. Without counting calories, without feeling hungry, excess fat will just slide off.

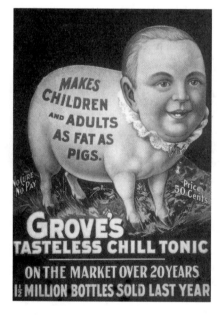

MAKES CHILDREN AND ADULTS AS FAT AS PIGS.

No cure No pay   Price 50 Cents

GROVE'S TASTELESS CHILL TONIC

ON THE MARKET OVER 20 YEARS 1½ MILLION BOTTLES SOLD LAST YEAR

Attitudes Change!

Cancer & the Immune System:

Current methods of treating cancer are rudimentary and barbaric. It is slowly being realized that it is far better to prevent cancer occurring in the first place. And the best prevention? That comes from the body itself! Over aeons, the immune system has developed the ability to search out and eliminate cancerous cells as they arise. Cells are going cancerous many times a minute. The immune system can cope with this load provided it is given the tools to do the job.

Too often the immune system is *malnourished* and operating like a misfiring auto engine. What nourishment does it need? It needs a range of micro-nutrients like minerals, vitamins, bioflavonoids, phenols and many other substances whose presence can only be suspected. All we know is that certain kinds of foods are helpful and others are not. Eating in certain ways is helpful, other ways are not.

Too often the immune system is *undermined* by tasks that should not be necessary. Tasks like sweeping up the débris from a malfunctioning gut, or the consumption of foods that depress the immune system.

Even when some cancers have established themselves, they are kept under control by an immune system that is operating at 100% efficiency. Eating naturally ensures that the full weight of the immune system is concentrated on the battle against cancerous cells.

Heart Disease, High Blood Pressure, and Atherosclerosis

These are leading killers in the United States, and they are totally preventable. These diseases were virtually unknown until 60 years ago. The rise has been inexorable since then. And their rise is in lockstep with the increased consumption of *meat, saturated fat* and *bad carbohydrates*. You don't even need to go back to a Stone Age diet to be sure of never dying of these diseases. Just go back to the way your grandparents used to eat.

The good news is that eating naturally will not only stop the progress of these diseases in their tracks, there is a good chance that some of the damage can be undone.

Constipation, Colon Cancer and Diverticulosis

These are all due to a state of chronic constipation brought about by an impoverished diet, low in fibre and high in foods that starve friendly bacteria. Eating naturally will banish constipation forever to a distant, unpleasant memory, and these intestinal diseases will be prevented. If diseases have already happened, they will be controlled and even regressed.

Strokes and Thromboses

There is no excuse for a stroke or a thrombosis happening before a very advanced age. They are provoked by the abnormal production of certain hormones like *thromboxane*, the powerful blood clotting hormone. One way in which we cause this abnormal production of 'bad' hormones is by the abnormal production of another hormone, insulin. And what is at the root of abnormal insulin production? The abnormal consumption of *bad carbohydrates.*

Whew! This is just one tiny example of how foods act like drugs and set in motion a complex chain of events that leads to ill health. And what are bad carbohydrates? You'll discover those when you get to Chapter Five. Just know that when you eat naturally, you don't produce abnormal quantities of thromboxane, or indeed any of the other illness-provoking 'bad' hormones.

Diabetes

Adult onset diabetes was a rare disease until about 50 years ago. Its incidence is growing geometrically and is expected to attain nearly 20% of the American adult population in 10 years time. It is responsible for most cases of blindness, amputations and kidney disease. Diabetes multiplies up the risk of mortality from cardio-vascular disease.

Diabetes has grown from nearly zero just 50 years ago to being a significant crippling and killing disease today.

Sample Bad Fats:

butter
margarine
cereal oils
(sunflower,
safflower,
peanut, corn)
animal fat
see Chapter Five,
What We Eat.

Sample Favourable Fats:

Canola oil
walnut oil
flax oil
fish oil
See Chapter Five.

Diabetes is another eminently preventable disease. One main cause of diabetes is the over-consumption of *bad* carbohydrates, including sugar. The rise in consumption of sugar per year has risen exponentially from zero 200 years ago (see chart in Chapter Four) to 130 lb./head today! This over-consumption of *bad* carbohydrates causes a massive insulin reaction. Over time, the pancreas' ability to function properly is wrecked, and the fat cells fail to function properly.

Worse, the abnormal quantities of insulin floating around in the bloodstream are causing havoc. Blood clots form, arteries harden, cholesterol is produced, the immune system is depressed, the kidneys fail, even the bones lose calcium!

Eating naturally will ensure that you never drive yourself into a state of diabetes, or if you already have it, control it in ways that will minimize damage to the body.

Rheumatoid Arthritis

The evidence is now conclusive that this agonizing and debilitating disease is provoked by an allergic reaction to some vector affecting the body's nerves. The nerves are tricked into falsely sending signals to cells in the joints to swell up. What could cause this? One major suspect is the release of bacteria and toxins into the bloodstream from a "leaky colon" and through a liver which is already too intoxicated to filter them out.

A second major suspect is the production of 'bad' eicosonoids. Eicosonoids are super-hormones which emerge, give their instructions and quickly disappear. 'Bad' eicosonoids are simply the ones which are produced in excess due to some unbalancing factor. One of these factors is an excess of insulin caused by *bad* carbohydrates.

A third major suspect is the consumption of 'bad' fats, particularly hydrogenated vegetable fats (present in margarine and many manufactured foods), and the absence of good fats in the diet, such as the Omega 3 series.

Whatever the trigger, rheumatoid arthritis has been found to be reduced or even miraculously cured, simply by changes to the diet. And what are those changes? Why ones which correspond to a way of Natural Eating!

Circulation and complexion

One of the most pleasing benefits of eating naturally is that the little capillaries in the face and extremities are kept flushed out and healthy. Fingers and toes remain warm and sensitive. The cheeks glow with good health.

Osteoporosis

Osteoporosis is a disease of the bone, and we have very good records of the condition of human bones going back tens of thousands of years. It is a condition virtually unknown by our Pleistocene ancestors. No bones there looking like Gruyère cheese. No friable, chalky vertebrae collapsing under their own weight.

And yet for all the calcium tablets swallowed, for all the milk being drunk, osteoporosis is reaching epidemic proportions! What is going wrong? It is due to the refusal to look at the root causes of osteoporosis. Only a few enlightened doctors draw the obvious conclusion that the reason our bones get to look like Swiss cheese is due to the way that we eat.

Contrary to popular myth, osteoporosis is caused by hormonal imbalances not calcium deficiency. It is a problem of our bodies not using the calcium that it is given properly. This flies in the face of 'conventional' wisdom. Doctors exhort us to consume ever increasing quantities of calcium tablets and calcium-rich products like milk.

Study after study shows that taking calcium tablets is about as useful as trying to fill the bathtub with a sieve without the bath plug! We need to eat in a way which puts the bath plug in place and which closes the holes of the sieve. Eating naturally does just that - just like it did for our Pleistocene ancestors.

Want to know how? Go to Chapter Eight, *The Food/Disease Connection*.

Digestion

The consumption of over-the-counter digestion remedies in Western Countries is at an all-time high. This is due, without any equivocation, to the appalling eating habits that prevail. Restructuring your eating habits so as to eat naturally will banish for ever the debilitating stomach upsets, acidity, cramps and nauseas that so many people are martyr to.

Case Histories

Does this all sound too good to be true? Here is a sample of the many people who have benefited from adopting the Natural Eating Pattern (their names have been changed to protect privacy.)

John

"I've had the first good night's sleep in 20 years!"

John, of Phoenix, Arizona, middle-aged and overweight, complained that he never got a good night's sleep. He always woke up in the middle of the night with heartburn and digestive disorder.

He had a classical American eating pattern, that is to say, anything goes. It was suggested that he try avoiding bad food combinations.

That very evening he went to a steak house. He started with a mixed salad. Then went on to a smaller steak than usual, accompanied by some vegetables. For dessert he had some fresh strawberries.

He avoided:

• *bad* carbohydrates generally

• choosing a protein or *bad* carbohydrate starter

• choosing a dessert containing starches such as apple pie or chocolate cake

He turned away:

• the bread rolls, the french fries and the wild rice (*bad* carbohydrates).

Instead of his customary beer, John drank a glass of dry red wine with the meal. He also drank some water.

This meal was a well-combined meal with plant food (salads and vegetables) dominating. To this was added just one protein, the steak. The quantity was modest. There were absolutely *no* bad carbohydrates. The dessert consisted of one of the two fruits that it is possible to eat at the end of a meal, strawberries. (The other is raspberry).

John called in the next morning ecstatic. He had just had the first good night's sleep in 20 years! From then on John was careful about his combinations and his body soon reminded him if he stepped out of line.

Levinia

"For the first time in 5 years I am free of Candida!"

Levinia, 10 pounds overweight and twenty-something, had been battling outbreaks of candida for many years. She suffered flare-ups of vaginal discharge with gastrointestinal upset, constipation, itching rectum, gas, cramps, and flu-like symptoms. Analysis had revealed candida spores in her blood. If this were true, there was no time to lose. Once candida generalizes throughout the body, the outlook is grim.

Levinia's doctor had prescribed the usual medications but they only seemed to have a temporary effect. She had heard in a Natural Eating seminar that candida is a common consequence of Western dietary errors. Levinia wanted to ensure that her eating patterns were helping rather than hindering her recovery.

Candida is a kind of yeast that is present in everyone's intestine. It is a malevolent organism, but under healthy conditions it is kept at bay by:

• the 'friendly' bacteria in the intestine which crowd out harmful organisms

- the immune system, which is patrolling the body gobbling up foreign bodies

Candida growth is encouraged by:

- the foods it likes, notably the undigested particles of sugars and starches
- the absence of 'friendly' bacteria in the intestine
- a weak immune system
- a porous intestine, that allows the yeast to grow and spread throughout the body
- high levels of sugar in the blood

Eating strictly 'naturally' would, of itself, be all that is necessary to bring candida under control. However, it was important that Levinia emphasize the measures that would help her particular condition. She was coached in the Natural Eating method with strict emphasis on practices that:

- reinforce her immune system
- starve the candida of nourishment
- ensure good intestinal health
- provide nourishment to 'good' bacteria

A while later, Levinia called, overjoyed. She had enjoyed a month without any of the horrible candida symptoms, felt a thousand times better... and as a bonus had lost 5 pounds in weight!

Robert

"I've taken off 45 pounds in four months!"

Robert, late 60s, dynamic businessman, had a large paunch. Measuring 5' 11" and weighing 240 pounds Robert had a Body Mass Index (BMI) of 34. According to the charts, this put him in the 'seriously-at-risk obese' category. Not surprisingly, Robert's doctor told him that if he wanted to live another twenty years, he should trim down as fast and as far as possible.

Robert had tried at various times to slim down, but always to no avail. The usual story: diets hard to keep up, constantly feeling hungry, weight back on within days.

Robert heard the Natural Eating philosophy expounded and it 'spoke to him'. Over a long week-end Robert and his wife were coached in all the subtleties of surviving in the 'Supermarket Jungle'.

Three months later Robert called in to say that he has just been to the tailor to have 6 inches taken out of the waist of his pants! Robert had lost

45 pounds. He had never eaten so much, had never felt hungry, and (tongue-in-cheek) had discovered the secret of the Natural Eating method – that you defecate a lot!

Robert still has a little way to go to attain his ideal weight of 180 pounds max. But Robert's general state of health is already 100% better. Most importantly, he has learned the new habits that will maintain his weight and health permanently.

Jason

"I'm over the moon! Last year I was treated for cancer. Since going on your program my immune system has been so reinforced that there is no more sign of cancerous cells. In addition my cholesterol and triglyceride levels are right down."

Jason, business tycoon, late 60s, tall and slim, rang in one day.

"You won't remember me, but I came to one of your seminars about three months ago. We had heard your radio show and what you said about the immune system suppressing cancer struck a chord with me.

I had finished conventional therapies for bladder cancer about a year ago. They had cleaned it up, but the three month check-ups showed that the cancer was still lying in wait.

We listened to you speak and, after initial skepticism my wife and I were won over to your precepts. We bought your 'Survival Manual', had a final dinner at a smart restaurant, looked at each other, and agreed that we would go on the program the next day.

I gave your manual to my chef and told him that from now on we were going to eat like this. My chef, who I had plucked out of the best Swiss school of cuisine, had culture shock. To his credit, he used his imagination to create meals that fit in so well with your program that our guests don't even notice!

Yesterday, my specialist doctor called with the results of the most recent tests. 'What on earth have you been doing!' he asked.

I replied nervously that I had only tried a new way of eating. I imagined that he had some awful news to communicate.

'Your test results are remarkable! Your triglycerides and cholesterol are right down, and best of all, no sign of pre-cancerous cells!'"

Jason remained clear of cancer and his vital signs remained good and improving.

Jason's wife was pleased too. Since abandoning bad carbohydrates, after three days of withdrawal, her brain had cleared "like a veil lifting." As an added bonus she had trimmed down 15 pounds to her ideal weight.

Genevieve

Genevieve, a statuesque lady in middle age, was consuming quantities of thick fluids from flasks that she pulled out of a capacious handbag. Genevieve was not eating any solids, simply drinking juiced vegetables and fruits all day long.

She explained that she suffered from irritable bowel syndrome and that this was the only way she knew to bring it under control. But as soon as she stopped, the symptoms would flare up again.

Allergies, irritable bowel, asthma, are always difficult to track down and fix. The triggers can be manifold and there are often non-nutritional factors as well. Nevertheless, the first thing to do if you find yourself in a hole is to stop digging! That is to say, stop doing the things that we know for sure are a problem to the body.

Irritable bowel is often an allergic reaction to some foodstuff. Almost always it is a foodstuff to which the body is not naturally adapted. The most common allergens are grains, (particularly wheat gluten) and dairy products.

Of course the Natural Eater would not eat much, if any of these foods, but to Genevieve this was a revelation. It is not only acceptable but positively helpful to eliminate these harmful 'novelty' foods in the human diet.

Genevieve tried eating naturally for a few weeks.

She contacted us a few weeks later to say:

"You have revolutionized my diet and health! When I stopped eating grains, amazing things happened – the irritable bowel went away after years of suffering."

———— ◆ ————

This is just a typical sample of those people who have benefited from getting their eating habits under control. They got their body biochemistry functioning in harmony with the way the body works.

One major theme of this book is this: You do not have to micromanage the way your body functions, indeed it is impossible! But if you give it the tools to do the job, then your body will do all the micromanagement necessary.

Another theme of this book is that, simply by adopting Natural Eating habits, your ability to control and develop good health will be assured right across the board. Genetically, you may have been dealt a good or a bad hand. Most people today play their hand badly! But good hand or bad hand, this book will tell you how to play that hand to best advantage.

———— ◆ ————

Play your hand well, not badly – it makes sense!

———— ◆ ————

C h a p t e r   T h r e e

The Human Story

How it was before

We know quite a lot about the location of the birthplace of the human race. Even in Victorian times, when the great apes, the chimpanzee and gorilla were first discovered in equatorial Africa, some researchers speculated that this too was the birthplace of mankind. Over the intervening years, fossil evidence came to light that reinforced this theory.

To the Near East and the rest of the world

AFRICA

Ethiopia

Kenya

Tanzania

Much more dramatically, in the last few years evidence has come from a totally new direction, DNA analysis. It is now clear that everyone on this planet is descended from a group of ancestors that lived in the savannahs of East Africa some 80,000 years ago. It even appears that we are all descended from just one woman who lived in the group 100,000 to 150,000 years earlier, the so-called 'Eve' hypothesis. There was not necessarily anything special about her. It's just that the bloodlines of all the other women of the tribe have petered out down the generations.

At that time the total world population of humans was probably no more than about 10,000. And how were they living? We can now get a good idea from a number of areas of research. For example, by studying such features as teeth and jaws, we know that they were designed for a particular kind of eating pattern. There are even studies of enamel thickness, tooth wear, micro-scratches and striations that can be matched with known patterns today.

There are studies of the vegetation that grew in the area at the time, and of the animal life that abounded. Calculations are made as to the most efficient use of energy expenditure to gain food. (It is assumed that, back then, our ancestors were no more inclined to work than we are today.) For example, hunting is a high energy expenditure with an uncertain reward. It is also risky. Rather than *getting* dinner, the hunter could finish up *as* dinner. Foraging for nuts, fruits, tubers, roots, flowers, edible gums, shellfish, caterpillars, was much surer, safer and *energy efficient.*

The forensic archaeologists can tell a lot from both human and animal bones. Early humans were tall: Turkana boy, only about 12 years old, would have grown to 6 feet. We can tell a lot about the diseases they suffered and didn't suffer. For example, osteoporosis, gallstones, kidney stones, arthritis and dental caries (cavities) were virtually unknown.

It is possible to tell something from the animal bones that are found at ancient human encampments. Were these animals killed by humans? If so, were they killed for food? Or were these animals killed by some other predator and only then butchered by humans? Or was the animal killed by a leopard and dragged to the same leafy spot occupied by humans 20 years previously?

Mostly it is impossible to know from a pile of animal bones, accumulating over millennia, who ate them, let alone what proportion of the diet they represent. After all, bones fossilize very well; vegetation doesn't fossilize at all.

Nevertheless, clever analysis can cast some light on what really happened. For example, prey bones often bear scratch marks. Some of them are from the teeth of the predator that killed them, some are the marks of a stone tool. Sometimes they occur together. It is possible to discern which came first, the lion's teeth marks, or the stone knife. The studies to date suggest that humans mostly chopped the meat after a predator had first killed it.

This is not surprising. Back then there were no real weapons, not even bows and arrows. All that Pleistocene humans had were sharp sticks, sharp stones and their bare hands. The savvy strategy to procure meat would be to fight off the hyenas and vultures for the carcass of an animal brought down by a specialist killer, such as a lion.

If humans were eating meat, how important a part did it play in their diet? And what was it like? There is still a vigorous debate over the first question. There were times of plenty and times of food stress. What is very clear is that humans were eating *animal matter* in significant quantities say 20% of their diet. But notice the words 'animal matter'. A large part of their consumption would have been made up of lizards, snakes, bugs, caterpillars, frogs, insects, shellfish, eggs, and, yes, small game and carrion.

There is less debate about the *nature* of this animal matter. There are three remarkable features about it:

• it was very low fat no more than 3% (as against 25% fat in modern beef).

• the fat was very low in saturated fat and high in 'essential fatty acids' (exactly the opposite of modern supermarket meats).

- the essential fatty acids were present in a well-defined ratio of linoleic acid to alpha linolenic acid. The range of this ratio varied within close limits of between 4:1 and 1:1. It transpires that this fatty acid profile is exactly the profile that we modern humans need too. In the average western diet this ratio is totally distorted at 32:1, and we know that this has harmful health effects. More of this in Chapter Five, *How and What We Eat*.

But let's look a little more at these essential fatty acids. They are so important that they used to be called vitamin F_1 (linoleic acid) and vitamin F_2 (alpha linolenic acid). All the other fatty acids that human biochemistry needs can be made by the body from these two.

But why these two fatty acids in particular? The body never had to learn how to make them. *They were always there in the diet.* They were in the plants that the herbivores ate, so they were there in the herbivores that the carnivores ate, and ultimately they became part of the carnivores too. Those fatty acids were omnipresent in the whole nutritional environment and in that ideal ratio range of between 4:1 and 1:1 to boot!

A similar phenomenon is found with vitamin C. Humans, along with most other primates, are the only creatures that cannot make vitamin C in their bodies. This is not a fault, it's just that our bodies never had to learn to make it. *Vitamin C was always present in the diet* from the fruits and vegetation.

The body's need for these three vitamins (C, F_1 & F_2) alone tells us a lot about our Pleistocene ancestors' eating patterns.

How exactly did our ancestors live all those generations ago? We are now able to piece together a clear picture. They lived in groups of 35 to 50 people - men, women and children together. This group would have a territory of 200 to 300 square miles that they defended fiercely from incursions by neighbouring groups. Within this territory they wandered.

> *A hunter-gatherer needs a range of about 5 square. miles to feed himself. The maximum population that the continental United States could support like that is 600,000 hunter-gatherers. Compare this to the current US population of some 260 million. There is no going back!*

These people had no clothes and no possessions. According to the availability of the food supply they camped and then moved on every day if need be. They had no permanent shelter. Each night they would hunker down under a bush and maybe pull some branches over into a make-shift shelter.

They had fire and used it for light, warmth, cooking meat, and for firing the bush to chase out small animals. These people didn't plant, didn't

Average of some 50 Wild Vegetable Foods consumed by foragers. Values for 2 kg		
Protein	g	82
Fat	g	56
Carb.	g	460
Fibre	g	62
Energy	kcal	2600
Calcium	mg	2000
Potassium	mg	9800
Sodium	mg	210
Vitamin C	mg	540

conserve, didn't save, but they did make a mess wherever they went! They didn't wash, smelled like pole-cats and lived in relative squalor. And yet they were healthy and had good longevity. They had few predators and were much more likely to be killed by warfare with neighboring groups. It has been estimated that their percentage casualties per year were as much as those of the German population during World War II.

It is thought that, much of the time, our early hominid ancestors fulfilled their basic protein needs just by consuming plant foods.

These peoples had a choice of *hundreds* of edible plants, a rich variety compared to the 30 or so found in today's supermarkets. The adjacent table itemizes some important nutrients found in a basket of just 50 forager plant foods.

Yes, *protein is in vegetables too!* 82 g of protein is plenty for the average adult. Better still, it is absorbed in small doses throughout the day. Not a sudden, calcium depleting, kidney-bashing, amino-acid rush as happens when a large steak is eaten. Indeed, on average, Americans consume twice the amount of protein thought advisable.

Not only is there plenty of protein, there is plenty of calcium, yet not a glass of milk in sight.

Potassium is very high by western standards and not a banana in sight either. (Bananas are native to Indonesia, not Africa.)

Sodium is good and low. After all, they had no added salt and no processed foods. Sodium intrinsic to the plant was the only sodium in the diet.

More interesting is the ratio of potassium to sodium – about 40:1. The potassium/sodium ratio is important to keep electrolytes balanced at the level of cell metabolism. Get it wrong, and the heart stops beating, nerves stop functioning and muscles shut down. Get this ratio wrong in the diet, and the body particularly the kidneys, is battling to straighten it out. Today's Western diet reverses the desirable ratio. It is now known that this chronic imbalance in the potassium/sodium ratio is a factor in many cardio-vascular diseases, such as stroke, high blood-pressure, cardiac arrest and inelastic arteries.

Note that our ancestor's high potassium intakes came from vegetation. And the low sodium levels from the absence of table salt.

As for *vitamin C*, see what a high level it is 540 mg. There is ample evidence that the official R.N.I. (Recommended Nutritional Intake) of 60 g is far too low. It is good enough to prevent scurvy, yes, but not good enough for optimum health. So here is another sign-post, our Pleistocene ancestors were in the habit of consuming some *five times* the quantity of vitamin C habitually consumed by Americans. We can be sure that if vitamin C is constantly in the food supply, the human body will come to depend on it. Today we fall far short of supplying that need.

Fibre content at 62 g. is some *five times* the norm for Americans. We can be sure that our Pleistocene ancestors never suffered from constipation, colon cancer or diverticulosis. Also note the quality of the fibre is not a rough, indigestible, cereal bran, it is all from fruit and vegetables high in heart-healthy soluble fibre. That's another straw in the wind – humans are designed for a high consumption of soluble fibre, not cereal fibre.

A word about tubers and potatoes. A large percentage of our ancestors' food supply came from vegetation that was prized out of the ground (with a digging stick) that is, roots, tubers, corms, bulbs etc. A little known, but common characteristic of all these foods is that they were all low glycemic[1]. The tubers had very little starch (instead they had low glycemic inulin). The potato is a novelty in the human diet. It is high in starch and is strongly glycemic and insulinemic[1], both harmful properties. Regrettably the potato, although botanically a tuber, cannot be classed with the plant foods to which humans are naturally adapted.

Finally, note the quantity of plant food consumed is some 2 kg. (4½ lb.). This is the *volume* of food that we are designed to eat. Today, we eat *less* volume, but much higher *calorie-dense* foods. This is another major reversal in our naturally adapted eating pattern. We can be sure that there are health consequences.

Thus for hundreds of millennia the pattern remained the same. The climate didn't change, the food supply didn't change, and our bodies didn't change. The eating patterns remained sensibly the same: fruits, nuts, berries, roots, vegetation and, yes, the occasional egg, insect, grub and small game animal.

This process went on down the millennia in a slow rhythm in which the evolution of man was sensibly in harmony with his slowly changing environment. His biochemistry was in *equilibrium* with the fuel furnished by his foraging . Like every other creature, he fed from what was *naturally* available. His body was *naturally adapted* to his food supply.

The main characteristics of this food supply were high volume, low calorie density, low fat, high in nutrients and micro-nutrients and it was low glycemic index (more of that later).

These ancestors of ours were very successful. They multiplied and spread out over the whole of Africa. By 50,000 years ago they were crossing the land bridges into Asia, Europe, Australia and finally the Americas. By about 15,000 years ago the world was filled up. They were still wandering

---

Our prehistoric ancestors did not eat:

- *Milk, cream, butter, cheese*
- *Bread, breakfast cereals, popcorn, spaghetti, pizza, rice...*
- *Vegetable oils,*
- *Farmed meat (saturated fat)*
- *Sugars (sugar, honey, maple syrup, malt, corn syrup....)*

The Pleistocene diet was:

- *high in volume*
- *low calorie density*
- *high in micro-nutrients*
- *high in fibre*
- *very low fat*
- *low glycemic*
- *low salt*

---

1 The blood-sugar raising power of a food is measured by its glycemic index. The insulin raising power of a food is measured by its insulin index. Both these matters are of the highest importance in human health and are treated in greater detail in Chapter Five, How and What We Eat.

foragers needing 200 to 300 square miles per group.

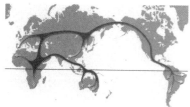

We can imagine the scene – still multiplying, groups becoming too large and needing to split up, but having nowhere to go except fight another group for its territory. Some groups found themselves in the most inhospitable and unlikely ecological niches, like the circumpolar Eskimos of the Arctic, and the Touareg of the pitiless Sahara Desert. Others, like the Polynesians, undertook ever more daring voyages to uninhabited islands. But inexorably, the world filled up and there was nowhere else to go.

Then one year, about 10,000 years ago, in a corner of what is now the borders of Turkey and Iraq, something extraordinary happened. A small band of these early foragers *took control* of their food supply. They stopped wandering and they *planted*. It meant staying in one place, protecting the crop, and inventing fences, hoes, drills, baskets and pots. It meant devising methods of *processing*, *conserving* and *storing* the crop. Finally, it meant inventing cooking. With these big changes coming such a short time ago in evolutionary terms, our bodies have not at all adapted to them.

Taking control of their food supply solved at a stroke the problems of overpopulation. Instead of 200 square miles, this group needed only 2 square miles to feed themselves. They had become farmers. This allowed much greater densities of population, and the growth of villages, towns, and cities. But there was a price to pay, as we shall see. Finally, over 6,000 years ago these peoples entered the eras of the great civilizations of Sumer, Egypt and Babylon. And that is where the history books begin.

This 'farming revolution' spread, during several thousand years, to almost every corner of the globe. That is to say that most peoples, all over the world, *took control* of their food supply, wherever they happened to be.

And, in taking control what happened? They cultivated not the crops that they were used to eating, but the crops that it was possible to cultivate. They favoured the crops that were easy to grow, protect, harvest, and store. That is, crops that were *convenient* and *practicable*.

As time went by, they also *domesticated* wild animals. Instead of the wide range of animal matter consumed before – caterpillars, locusts, ants, lizards, snakes and small game – they bred and raised a much *smaller variety* of *very different* animals, the cattle, sheep, pigs and fowl of today. These animals were chosen only because no other creature could be domesticated.

For the first time man started eating two kinds of new food: carbohydrates with high glycemic index, and meats high in saturated fat. In addition, some tribes, the Mongolian nomads and Aryan pastoralists in particular, introduced *dairy products*. For the first time too, man started cooking in a big way.

As the societies became richer, they could afford to be more frivolous. They cultivated crops and raised domesticated animals that were *tasty*, *prestigious*, and *amusing*.

Such is the progress of this trend that, today we eat foodstuffs almost exclusively because they are *convenient, tasty, cheap* and *attractive*. We have lost all touch with the eating patterns for which our bodies were designed.

——————— ◆ ———————

Today, we have lost touch with the eating patterns for which our bodies were designed.

——————— ◆ ———————

Evolutionary History tells us that our pre-historic diet contained
soft vegetation, fruit, nuts, insects, flowers, gums, some egg and some small game.

It did not contain
seeds, grains or cereals, dairy products, farm meat, saturated fat or vegetable oils.

That is a synopsis of what we understand about our pre-historic ancestors. This information can be compared to what we know about peoples who still lived in the same way in recent memory.

The great European explorations and expansion of the last few centuries put an end to the few extant forager lifestyles. Acculturation by contact with the West changed these primitive peoples' way of life forever.

Nevertheless, it has been possible to piece together historical accounts for some of the early contacts. For example, until 200 years ago, the Australian Aborigine still lived the foraging life-style. This applied to the whole continent – the size of the U.S. – which stretched from the cold temperate regions of Tasmania to the tropics of Queensland and the Northern Territories. It is estimated that even though the continent was filled to saturation, there were no more than 800,000 Aborigines.

The first European colonists of Australia were English convicts sentenced to 'transportation.' Some of them escaped from captivity and lived wild with the aboriginals. Later, their experiences were recorded by researchers. Other evidence comes from the first pioneers and missionaries to the 'outback'. They observed the aboriginals as they pushed back the frontier. Later researchers have worked with semi-traditional Aborigines to download their remembrances of times past.

All these accounts are helpful and point in the same direction. However, we must also recognize that these accounts were gathered under unscientific conditions and that as such, they have to be treated with more caution.

Similar remarks apply to other pre-farming peoples such as the Eskimo and the Plains Indians.

Attempts have been made in recent years to study so-called hunter-gatherer tribes like the Ache of Paraguay and the Bushmen of Southern Africa. 'So-called', because they have been influenced by proximity to the modern world, and they inhabit marginal ecological niches untypical of our hunter-gatherer forebears. Even so, useful and indicative data are obtained by researching them. There is not the space to discuss these data here, but there are several useful references in the bibliography.

Pre-farming peoples

The Australian Aborigine

The Australian Aborigine was the archetypal Pleistocene-type forager (or in common parlance 'hunter-gatherer'). His lifestyle has been closely studied. He was wise enough to never adopt agriculture, although he knew about the techniques from visiting Asian fishermen. The Australians lived in small groups of about 35 to 50 souls who wandered their territories of 200 to 350 square miles.

Traditional Aborigines had no clothes and no dwellings. Every night they pulled together a rough shelter out of branches. They carried with them virtually nothing. Everything was improvised for the occasion. Their few possessions were multifunctional and portable. Spears, woomeras[2] and boomerangs for the men. Digging sticks and grindstones for the women. Always, the band carried a "firestick," a flaming brand to set the campfire at night and fire the bush on occasion to trap animals. They were quite careless about this. Sometimes whole regions went up in smoke, simply to force out a small animal 50 feet away.

The Healthy Hounzas

Some of the healthiest and long-lived communities in the world are tribes that live simply, often in difficult circumstances. The Hounzas, for example, have excited interest ever since a young British Raj Army medical doctor, Robert McCarrison, had charge of them in a remote valley in the High Himalayas. They led a frugal life, cultivating root and vegetable crops and some apricot trees. Meat and dairy products formed only 1.5% of their diet.

McCarrison was astonished to find that the Hounzas suffered from no chronic diseases, that they had vigorous, muscular bodies to an advanced age, and degenerative diseases were unknown. They kept their teeth intact for life; that they had an extraordinary resistance to infections; the men were still procreating at the age of 75, and apparently lived to 100 years old.

*That was in 1904. McCarrison was so impressed that he monitored these people for another 14 years before returning to London. He found it difficult to believe, but after eliminating all other possibilities, reluctantly came to the conclusion that diet was the determining factor. He became a prestigious research scientist and was one of the first nutritionists to make himself unpopular by suggesting that **white bread, sugar, meat and dairy products** were at the origin of the average Londoner's comparative bad health.*

---

2 A hooked wooden stick used for launching a spear with greater force than can obtained by the arm alone.

The early settlers imagined, falsely, that the aboriginal life was incredibly hard. But even in the Great Central Desert, the aboriginal had a wide variety of plant and animal foods. This was demonstrated most spectacularly and tragically by the fate of the exploring party of Burke and Wills[3]. Having traversed the continent from south to north with a huge baggage train, they finally ran out of food and pack animals in the deserts of the return leg. They tried to live off the land as the aboriginals did, but without their detailed knowledge, they grew weaker. Wandering groups of Aborigines came across them and gave them some help, showing them how to pound seeds into a cake called "nardoo" for example. The explorers ate lots of it, but became ever weaker. They ate no vegetation – they just couldn't find any tomatoes, lettuce or onions!

The explorers were dying not from starvation but from *malnutrition*. They developed scurvy and other deficiency diseases. Burke and Wills died, but a third member of the party, King, was luckier. He was found by a group of Aborigines and he went to live with them. This time, he ate the full range of foods available to the Aborigine, none of which was a 'proper' food in European eyes. King survived and was rescued by a search party two months later.

All the evidence suggests that, just as for the Great Desert Aboriginal, our Pleistocene ancestors in East Africa could survive with a great deal of security in even the most hostile environments. There were plenty of fall-back positions. If certain favored foods were not available, then there were always others. And anyway, it was always possible to move on to another place where there would be yet another range of potential foods.

It is now believed that famine was an extremely rare occurrence amongst hunter-gatherers; they just had too many options. Famine is a phenomenon that came with the farming revolution. One single crop failure could wipe out a whole people. All their eggs, as ours are today, were in too few baskets.

What about the children? Infants were breast-fed 'on demand' until the age of at least three years and sometimes four. Solids were only introduced when the child had teeth to masticate properly. In the absence of processed foods and formula milk, it could only be that way. Weaning was started with suitably easy foods like the soft fatty meat from the tail of a goanna[4].

> *The aborigine's feeding pattern changed day to day and season to season. Sometimes their diet was high in vegetation with fruits such as 'bush raisins', 'bush tomatoes', 'quandong', 'bush plum', 'mulga apple', 'bloodwood apple', 'wild orange', 'red apple', 'cheesefruit', 'bush fig'; and vegetation such as water lilies, cycad, palm shoots, pandanas nut, gall nut, truffles, bush yams and innumerable edible leaves and roots.*

3 In the early days of European colonization of Australia, many exploring expeditions were mounted. One of the most celebrated, and most tragic is the expedition of Burke and Wills, sponsored by the Royal Society of Victoria. Burke left Melbourne with a party of 18 in August 1860 to explore the continent of Australia from Melbourne in the South to the Gulf of Carpentaria in the North. Impatiently, about half way up, he decided to leave 12 members behind at a base camp at Barcoo Creek, and continue with just three others. Burke and Wills died of malnutrition. Gray had already died 'of exhaustion' earlier in the return leg. Compare this amateurish bungling to the superb organization, professionalism and sensitive bush skills of the Lewis and Clark exploration of the American North West.

4 A large Australian monitor lizard.

The Aborigine, like most hunter-gatherers, exploited sources of food that were not available to other primates – roots and tubers. There was little competition from other mammals for these foodstuffs and, in hard times, they often provided the bulk of the diet. Indeed the women's digging stick has been called the aborigine's most important survival implement.

Most of the plant foods were eaten raw, although some would be baked in the ashes of the fire.

At other times, animal matter was important: witchetty grubs, locusts, lizards, snakes, goannas, magpie geese, eggs and, in coastal areas, turtles, shellfish and file snakes.

Sometimes there was a major kill of a kangaroo, emu, wallaby or, in coastal areas, barramundi, catfish, saratoga and dugong. This was a time of feasting when up to 25 pounds would be consumed at a sitting.

Mostly, animal matter was eaten cooked. Small game, snakes, lizards, grubs and bugs would be cooked whole in the embers of the fire. Larger animals would be eviscerated and the offal baked and eaten separately. Animal would be either baked whole or baked dissected. Meat was eaten 'rare'.

> **The Traditional Aborigine diet is:**
>
> • *high in volume*
> • *high in micro-nutrients*
> • *high in fibre*
> • *very low fat*
> • *low glycemic*
> *Sounds familiar?*

In times of scarcity, the millstone was pressed into service. The tedious business started of collecting grass seeds, winnowing, threshing, pounding and grinding. It was so labour intensive that the aboriginal did it only in times of dire need. In common with other cereals, the resulting flour had to be cooked to make it digestible. No pots or pans, just mix the flour with some water, form it into a patty and bake it in the embers of the camp fire. Those Aborigines who ate this way too often, had worn and pitted teeth.

The aboriginal had a sweet tooth. A disproportionate amount of his time went into searching for 'sweetmeats'. Honey ants (ants gorged with the nectar of flowers) were a favourite. In addition there was lerp (sweet insect secretion on eucalyptus leaves), blossoms and gums. If he was really lucky he would find a nest of honey bees to smoke out. But these were rare occasions and the amounts were small.

The traditional aboriginal was very lean but healthy. His Body Mass Index was 13.5 to 19. Compare this to the official US figure for healthy B.M.I. of 20 to 25. The Western target for body leanness is still relatively plump.

The aboriginal blood pressure, cholesterol and triglycerides were low. He had good (high) serum levels of hemoglobin, vitamin B12, vitamin C and folate. Atherosclerosis was rare. Diabetes was unknown.

All this came to an abrupt end when the European colonists arrived some 200 years ago. Very quickly the aboriginal became 'acculturated'. Flour, sugar and rice were distributed to the aboriginals by well-meaning mission stations. Sugar was eagerly sought. Consumption rose to 12 pounds per head per week.

Soon, tinned meat, tinned fruit, biscuits, confectionery and jam joined the list – to say nothing of alcohol and tobacco.

What has happened to the aboriginal's health? He now has very high rates of obesity, atherosclerosis, diabetes, dental caries, and ischemic heart disease. His life expectancy has dropped to 20 years less than his Caucasian counterparts.

Trials have been made where aboriginals suffering from these degenerative diseases were returned to traditional life patterns. Almost miraculously, within the space of weeks, their health returned.

The aboriginal has traded his calorie-poor, nutrient-dense diet for exactly the opposite: a calorie-dense, nutrient-poor diet. And he did this with alacrity. It is a lesson for all of us that our instincts in matters of nutrition cannot be trusted.

———— ◆ ————

Our instincts in matters of nutrition cannot be trusted!

———— ◆ ————

Native Americans

A similar fate awaited many other peoples when they came into contact with western dietary habits. In the United States, the Native Americans suffer in a similar way. Rates of obesity, diabetes and cardiovascular disease are much higher in this population. The much studied Pima Indians of Arizona have one of the highest rates of these diseases in the land. Trials with Navajo Indians have shown that when they return to traditional tribal patterns of eating, all their health indicators return to normal. Blood pressure, diabetes, obesity are all controlled.

The Eskimo

The Eskimo is an example of a race which lives in the most extreme of unpropitious environments. With virtually no vegetation and winter temperatures dropping to below -40° F, the eskimo lived out the greater part of his life eating fish, seal and whale. In spite of that, he had low blood pressure and low rates of heart disease. He got his vitamins from eating the skin of the seal and the stomach contents (lichens and mosses) of the caribou. He ate every part of the animal – brains, intestines, blood, even the feces. Almost always it was eaten raw. Living above the tree line, a campfire was a rare luxury.

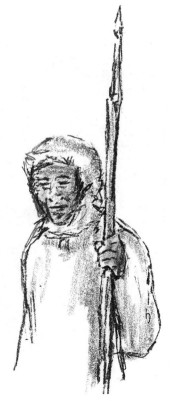

He cut off the blubber from his kill (seals, whales etc.) for use as lighting oil and other external uses. Seal and whale meat share similar characteristics with our ancestral wild game. There is little fat in the muscle meat (little 'marbling'), and it is particularly rich in essential fatty acids. As if that were not enough, the Eskimo high fish diet gave him eicosapentanoic acid – a great heart protector.

In fact it was perhaps too much of a good thing. Typically Eskimo bleeding time was high, and they suffered from difficult-to-stop nosebleeds.

We can learn something too from his high calcium intake of up to 2,000 mg/day. In spite of this mega-dose of calcium, the Eskimo suffered bone demineralisation and *osteoporosis.* Isn't this counter-intuitive? Today, we know that the culprit is the *high meat diet.* (The mechanisms are discussed in Chapter Eight.)

The Eskimo is an example of a race which lived successfully enough with very little in the way of fruit and vegetable in the diet. Nevertheless, his life expectancy was low – around 50 years. The Eskimo died of accelerated ageing.

Today, with Westernization, the Eskimo has suffered the same fate as the other hunter-gatherers. He suffers from obesity, heart disease, diabetes and high mortality. Life expectancy has dropped even lower, to around 35 years.

Hunter-gatherer studies tell us that a favorable diet contained
**soft vegetation, fruit, nuts, insects, flowers, gums,
some egg, some seafood and some game.**

It did not contain
**seeds, grains or cereals, sugars, dairy products, farm meat,
saturated fat or vegetable oils, salt.**

Forensic Archaeology

Forensic archaeology is the science of detecting and deducing from archaeological remains. For example, skeletons and their habitats are analyzed for various periods in human history. Forensic archaeologists can deduce a surprising amount from these remains.

The Dwarfing of the Human Race.

One clear and easy result is the comparison of skeletons today and in pre-farming times. Our Pleistocene ancestors had an average height some 6 inches greater than their descendants who took up farming. Today, in the opulent but still malnourished West, we have recovered only about 4 inches of the deficit. Maybe this comes as a surprise to read this. We do not realize how much our impression of past standards of living are highly conditioned by our image of life in the Victorian cities of the industrial revolution. Dickens and Hugo did such a good job in drawing attention to the wretched conditions that, even today, those images linger in our subconscious.

We have made huge progress since the nadir reached in the times of Dickens, but we are still a way from regaining the healthy lifestyle conditions enjoyed by our pre-farming Pleistocene ancestors. The only reason stopping us, in these times of plenty, are our own poor feeding choices.

———— ◆ ————

The reality is that farming radically changed our ancestors' eating patterns for the worse.

The responsibility is now within our own grasp to make wise feeding choices.

———— ◆ ————

The whole of recorded history is a story of the struggles of populations for 'living room'. There was always more population than land to support them. This did drive the incredible progress in extracting more and more food from the same land. But there was always a time lag.

Furthermore, under these pressures, humans were spreading into lands and climates for which they were not at all adapted. It is a great tribute to their ingenuity that farmers scratched a living in Northern Europe. But scratching was all it was. Our ancestors over the past couple of thousand years were in general malnourished - much more than their ancestors of 10,000 years earlier.

———— ◆ ————

Our recent ancestors were malnourished compared to our Pleistocene forebears.

———— ◆ ————

The Ancient Egyptians ate:

Fruits: apple, carob, christ's thorn, egyptian plum, fig, grape, hegelig, juniper, olive, argun palm, date palm, persea, pomegranate, sycamore fig, water-melon and many more.

Vegetables: garlic, onion, radish, turnip, bulbs, agrostis, celery, cress, leek, lettuce, purslane, goats beard, saffron, water chestnut, cucumber, okra, gourd, and many more.

Legumes: beans, chick pea, lentil, lupine, pea and vetch.

Animal Matter: ox, sheep, boar, heron, Nile perch and many more.

Ancient peoples benefited from:

- *fruits, vegetables and nuts*
- *wild game and fowl in moderation*

Ancient peoples suffered from:

- *bread, honey,*
- *farmed meat*

Ancient peoples did not consume:

- *milk, butter, cheese*
- *corn oil, sunflower oil, safflower oil*

The Drudgery of Early Farming:

Analysis of the skeletons of those who took up farming, shows that they must have done it under considerable duress. It was that, or die of famine. Their skeletons show signs of *osteo-arthritis, carpal tunnel syndrome, and collapsed vertebrae.* Why was this? It was due to the drudgery of grinding grains, from morning till night, between two slabs of stone. And, in view of the bone deformities that they suffered, even the youngest children were pressed into service. In pre-historic times no one lived on grains from choice.

———————— ◆ ————————

In pre-historic times no one lived on grains from choice!

———————— ◆ ————————

Early Nutritional Diseases:

We have extensive evidence from early Sumerian and Egyptian sites over 4,000 years ago. It is quite remarkable that the Ancient Egyptians have left us a legacy of sumptuous burial tombs (the pyramids) with inscriptions of their daily life. As a bonus they left the embalmed mummies, accompanied by daily artifacts, for us to analyze.

Even the ordinary folk, who were simply buried in the sand outside the cities, have been preserved by the dryness of the environment. We therefore know quite a lot about their state of health too.

Typically populations, as they developed farming, gradually developed degenerative diseases. The wealthy Pharaohs of Egypt, gorged themselves *on bread, honeyed cakes, ox, game, fowl, fruits, figs, dates, wine and beer.* Not surprisingly, they suffered from *obesity, atherosclerosis, diabetes, and gallstones.*

We know that the ordinary people, who typically ate vegetables, rough whole bread, olive oil and figs, were on the whole lean and healthy. However, all classes suffered from *gum disease, dental cavities and abscesses.* This is put down to the high consumption of bread. All classes suffered worn and pitted teeth from the high grit content of the flour.

All classes suffered too from parasites such as guinea worm and river blindness. The Egyptian civilization was particularly vulnerable, being built upon the Nile with its regular floods.

As techniques 'improved' for making bread lighter, and the taste for whiter bread became popular, so dental cavities (caries) made its first appearance. Dental caries was virtually unknown in the times before the invention of bread.

On the other hand there is a notable absence of diseases such as *syphilis, cancer, tuberculosis* and *rickets*. This gives us pause for thought. How is it that not one of the tens of thousands of mummies examined shows signs of cancer? The answer will come later in the book, but we can be sure that the predominant reason is that some aspect of the ancient Egyptian diet was protective.

Studies of Early Civilizations show that:

- Fruit, vegetables, salads, nuts, some fish are helpful.
- Farm meat, saturated fat, dairy products, vegetable oils, refined cereals, sugars, are harmful.

Epidemiological (Population) Studies

Mankind has shown immense adaptability and ingenuity as he has spread out all over the globe. He has had to live under conditions to which he is not at all adapted. It is like a vast laboratory where a multitude of different experiments are going on simultaneously. We can analyze the different lifestyles and compare them to the health consequences that result.

In the last few decades, the eating habits of whole populations have been studied. Links have been sought between these habits and the measured incidence of various diseases and illnesses.

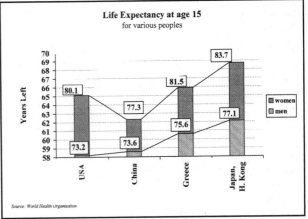

This graph of Life Expectancies for a variety of countries throws up a number of interesting points:

- American men have the lowest life expectancy of the countries shown
- Chinese men have a higher life expectancy than Americans – even though in China the means of keeping old people alive for many years simply don't exist.

- Chinese men, when they migrate to Hong Kong (HK) where medical support is to Western standards, have the longest life expectancy in the world. (Hong Kong is almost entirely populated by recent Chinese migrants.)

- Women live longer than men.

• The Japanese have, with the Hong Kongers, just about the longest life expectancies in the world.

It is statistics like this these give epidemiologists plenty to ponder.

The Japanese

Japanese men have a life expectancy 4 years greater than Americans. *But only on condition that they stay in Japan.*

When Japanese migrate to America and adopt the American 'way of life' including its diet, their life expectancy drops to the American norm and they get the same diseases.

At home, by a fluke of culture, geography and good luck, they have hit on a good eating pattern. (See box). But even so, it is not perfect. For example, the Japanese high consumption of salt (in soy sauce) gives them a high rate of death from stroke.

The Japanese traditionally consume rice as a staple. Rice is 'empty calories' having a low micro-nutrient and low protein content. Rice's glycemic index, however, is better than Western staples (wheat and corn) and falls in the 'Borderline' category. The Japanese regard rice as being a low quality 'filler' (which it is) and feel bad about serving up large quantities of it. Unknowingly this cultural pressure is health-helpful as is its substitution by plant food where possible.

Traditionally, the Japanese are Buddhists, and as such they do not eat meat. However, they do eat fish. So by chance, they discard a harmful foodstuff and pick on a helpful one. Even so, they do make one mistake, they often eat the fish raw. As a result, the Japanese suffer significantly from various intestinal worms and parasites.

> *The Japanese incidence of the following ailments is a tiny fraction of that for Americans: heart disease, colon cancer, prostate cancer, breast cancer, diabetes, high blood pressure*
>
> *The Traditional Japanese diet is rich in vegetables and fruits. It contains: little or no meat; some fish; some rice has no dairy products and is extremely low fat.*

The Cretans

Similar observations have been made with the peoples of the Mediterranean northern rim. The Cretans, (whose statistics boost the Greek life expectancies in the graph) had one of the highest life expectancies in the world, in spite of a hard lifestyle.

This so-called 'Cretan' or 'Mediterranean diet' has gained a lot of currency, and rightly so. Its *consumption profile* is much closer to the ideal for human beings.

Note that this so-called Mediterranean diet contains no spaghetti, pizza or medallions de veau. Coincidentally, the

> *The Cretan incidence of heart disease, colon cancers, high blood pressure , and diabetes are all much lower than in the Northern peoples of Europe and of the Americas.*
>
> *How do Cretans eat?*
> *fruit and vegetables - plenty*
> *rough ground bread - some*
> *fish - some*
> *goat's cheese - some*
> *meat, sugar, pastry - little or none*
> *milk, cream, butter, vegetable oil - none.*
> *They drink: wine in moderate quantities.*

Cretans use an oil (olive) that is neutral in its health impact. Less well known is their high consumption of *purslane*. This is a plant that used to be well known both in Europe and in North America. What is so special about it? It has a remarkably high alpha-linolenic acid content. The full significance of this is explained in Chapter Five. Again, by chance, the Cretans have hit upon a plant food that supplies the essential fatty acid, vitamin F_2 (alpha-linolenic acid) in which the average Westerner suffers a deficiency.

Sadly, with the advance of prosperity and the crumbling of old traditions, both the Japanese and the Cretans are adopting Western eating habits. The deterioration in their health is now being documented.

Clinical Trials

Literally thousands of clinical trials have been carried out to test various hypotheses about food and its physiological effects. A sample is given below:

The Lyon Diet Heart Study

A group of 606 heart attack patients living in Lyon, France, was divided into a control group and an experimental group. The control group carried on eating as before a diet typical of Western industrial societies.

The experimental group was told to adopt a Cretan type diet:

More green vegetables, more root vegetables, more fish, less meat (replace beef, pork and lamb with poultry), *no day without fruit*, and replace butter and cream with a special margarine made from canola oil. All other fats were replaced by olive oil and/or canola oil. Moderate wine consumption was allowed.

Lyon Diet Heart Study		
Cardiovascular Deaths	Control (Western)	Test (Cretan)
Sudden deaths	8	0
Other deaths	8	3
Total deaths	**16**	**3**
Non fatal heart attack	**17**	**5**
Cretan diet saves French lives		

After 27 months the death rate of the experimental group was so dramatically lower than the control group, that the experiment was stopped early so that the control group could benefit from this knowledge.

All this is to do with the Cretan or 'Mediterranean' diet. It is a way of eating which is demonstrably heart healthy. Yet there are other organs and diseases to consider and, as we shall see later, there are some significant improvements that are still to be made.

Summary of Clinical Trials

Thousands of similar clinical studies have been carried out. The main lessons are distilled into these schedules:

Helpful Foodstuffs		
Foodstuff	**Harmful Effects**	**Diseases Inhibited**
fruits vegetables salads tubers berries nuts (moderation) fish, oily (moderation) wild animal matter (moderation)	NONE	cancers heart disease high blood pressure infectious diseases bowel diseases constipation indigestion diabetes obesity arthritis osteoporosis

Harmful Foodstuffs		
Foodstuff	**Harmful Effects**	**Helpful Effects**
farm meat dairy products saturated fats bulk vegetable oils sugars starches	cancers obesity heart disease osteoporosis constipation indigestion allergies auto-immune diseases infectious diseases high blood pressure stroke	NONE

Doesn't this seem familiar? And isn't it extraordinary that there is no disease that can be imputed to a high plant food diet? The full impact of these helpful/harmful foodstuffs on health is documented in Chapter Eight, *The Food/Disease Connection.*

Creatures With Human-Like Body Plans

Another helpful tack is to look at creatures who are built to similar body plans to ours. These creatures are the class known as primates, the great apes being the most like us. From DNA analysis we now know that we share over 98.0% of our genes with both the chimpanzee and the gorilla. Our basic anatomy and biochemistry are almost identical.

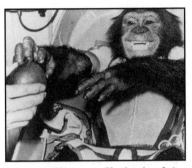

Astronaut Chimpanzee 'Ham' grabs a fruit. He looks pleased to return to Earth after his Mercury space-flight. Ham was pioneering for Alan Shepherd.

Courtesy: NASA

For these reasons researchers, after they have first tested mice and guinea pigs, try a new drug on a chimpanzee for a final check. If it works on him, and is harmless to him, then that is the nearest proof possible that it will be fine for humans too.

It is by studying the great apes, that we can learn a lot about how human bodies work, too.

The great apes live in tropical rain forests and eat what they find there. Tropical rain forests don't have marked seasons. Vegetation can be flowering, fruiting, seeding and regenerating at any time of the year.

Nevertheless, there is a rhythm of drier and rainier seasons which means that there are times of plenty and times of food stress.

The great apes have a very wide territory and they roam around it like nomads foraging for food. Every night they make a nest in the trees out of branches bent and broken into place. Great apes are messy creatures leaving excreta and debris as they go. Being forest nomads, they have never had to develop a sense of neat housekeeping.

The Opportunistic Chimpanzee

We know that chimpanzees have social structures similar to ours. They have family quarrels, power struggles, intrigues, alliances, deviousness and loyalty and devotion.

From studies in the wild we know how they eat. They live in tropical African forests and they are still partly tree dwelling. Chimpanzees eat what they find in trees. That is to say fruit (mostly), vegetation, flowers, gums, nuts and berries. They will opportunistically eat all kinds of things if they come across them: birds' eggs, grubs, termites and other bugs. The Chimpanzee is a curious creature, ready to try most things, but also quite fussy. He will inspect his food carefully, removing any offending part before consuming it.

Chimpanzees will occasionally even hunt small mammals such as infant monkeys. They hunt as a team, corner the monkey and then, between them, kill the monkey by tearing it limb from limb. Unlike true carnivores, chimpanzees *don't have* (as humans don't have), naturally endowed

Typical Day's Consumption in Captivity 400 lb. Gorilla			160 lbs. Human
Foodstuff	Amount	English	Grams
lettuce	3 heads	3 lbs.	480
celery	3 bunches	6 lbs.	1,000
apples	6 items	1.5 lbs.	250
oranges	6 items	2 lbs.	320
bananas	3 items	1.5 lbs.	250
carrots	3 items	1 lbs.	160
kale	3 bunches	6 lbs.	1,000
cantaloupe	1 item	3 lbs.	480
nuts	4 oz	4 oz	40
raisins	8 oz	8 oz	80
corn	8 oz	8 oz	80
pecans	4 oz	4 oz	40
sweet potato	3 items	1 lb.	160
tomato	2 no	0.5 lb.	80
Totals		26.5 lbs.	4.5 kgs. (10 lb.)

For comparison purposes, the quantities are scaled down for a 160 pound human. Even so it represents ten pounds of food intake per day. Humans are not gorillas and it is not suggested here that we should slavishly model our eating patterns on them. All the same, humans can and do eat like that and vegans can draw inspiration from this vegan feeding pattern. They should replace much of that pasta, bread, potato and cereals by high micro-nutrient density plant food.

killing weapons such as needle sharp teeth or razor claws.

These hunting expeditions are rare occurrences and had never been observed until the 1960s. They happen at a precise season of the year and seem to be linked to male power struggles and the seduction of females. At such times, the percentage of meat rises to 30 – 40 % of the diet. There are other periods of the year when no meat is consumed at all. Averaged over the year, it has been estimated that 90% of a chimpanzee's diet is vegetable matter, with a high emphasis on fruit.

Chimpanzees range widely to obtain their food, particularly up and down mountainsides, to get a variety of vegetation from the different altitude zones. They go out of their way to do this, as though they know that their nutrients are not to be found in just one spot.

The Stolid Gorilla

The gorilla is a total vegetarian. Although an adult male weighs 400 pounds of solid bone and muscle, he lives entirely on the fruits and vegetation found in the tropical rain forest. A gorilla will not eat bird's eggs should they be right next to him.

The gorilla gets all his nutrients from what he eats, chiefly vegetation, what we would call leafy green vegetables and salads. His diet also includes nuts, flowers, mature leaves, twigs, and gums. Protein comes entirely from the vegetation; energy from the carbohydrates in the fruit and vegetation; vitamins and minerals (including calcium and iron) are all present in perfectly healthy quantities.

Look at the adjacent table. It is the food typically consumed in a day by a gorilla in captivity. This particular menu has been chosen because it contains only foods that humans eat too. That gives a direct comparison with what a human might consume on such a typical day. In practice, over a period of time, a gorilla will be eating, even in a zoo, a huge range of plant foods including gums, flowers, branches and twigs.

In the wild, the gorilla would not be eating raisins, sweet potatoes, or corn. The zookeeper clearly has not heard of the Natural Eating Pattern! In mitigation, note that these non-primate foods form only a small proportion of the total intake.

The gorilla ranges less widely than the chimpanzee. He is less fussy and is more of a slow-moving vegetation processor. With all that food he has got to eat, he just keeps stuffing down whatever is closest to hand.

A fully grown male gorilla, although a vegan vegetarian, weighs 400 lb. of solid bone and muscle.

The Great Ape Diet Summarized

The chief characteristic of the great ape diet is that it is high in volume, low in calorie density, rich in micro-nutrients; high in fibre and very low in fat. There are no cereals, dairy products, bulk fats or oils, fish, or starches. There is virtually no meat. Sound familiar?

The great apes spend quite a lot of time eating, up to 30% of their waking time, even more for the gorilla. Their eating pattern is to start foraging in late morning and then 'graze' at regular intervals. That is to say, they eat little but often. But it is worth repeating, they are snacking on low calorie-density foods. If proof is needed, they hardly ever drink. The water content of their foodstuffs is greater than 80%. At this level the great ape can maintain a positive water balance without consuming water.

The Great Ape Diet:

- *high volume*
- *low calorie density*
- *rich in micro-nutrients*
- *very low fat*
- *low glycemic*

Sound familiar?

The Natural Eating Pattern

When we look at all these sources of evidence, and "connect the dots", we get the picture of the *naturally* adapted eating pattern – the pattern of eating appropriate to the human species:

The Naturally Adapted Eating Pattern is:

• *High Volume*
• *High Fibre*
• *Low Calorie Density*
• *High Micro-nutrient Density*
• *Low Glycemic*
• *Low Fat*
• *Low Salt*

The Naturally Adapted Eating Pattern is to:

• *eat little but often*
• *only start eating in the morning when ready*
• *eat lightly or not at all in the evening*

The Naturally Adapted Eating Pattern does Contain:

• *Vegetable matter (salads and vegetables) - lots*
• *Fruit - lots*
• *Low starch tubers, roots*
• *Wild Animal Matter - moderately*
• *Nuts - some*
• *Pulses - little or none*

The Naturally Adapted Eating Pattern does not Contain:

• *Cereals (wheat, bread, corn, rice, pasta, breakfast cereals, etc.)*
• *Vegetable Oils (sunflower, corn, safflower, peanut, palm oil, etc.)*
• *Dairy Products*
• *Farm Meat (beef, lamb, pork etc.)*
• *Sugars (sugar, malt, malto-dextrin, maple and corn syrup, honey, etc.)*

What does this mean in practical terms? After all, our ancestors walked barefoot. They also never washed and lived in what seems to us great squalor. Are we expected to return to that? Of course not.

The whole point about Natural Eating is that we learn the lessons. Lessons about the genetic programming that determines the harmonious eating pattern for our bodies. We can identify those aspects that are important and those which we can steer around. In other words we can prioritize.

And just because a food is new to the diet, doesn't mean that it is condemned out of hand. It just has to prove itself before it can be admitted to the club. For example, legumes, tomatoes, cocoa and even alcohol (under carefully controlled circumstances) get their 'Green Cards'.

The job of the next part of this book is to illustrate how this can be done. How we can get closer to our naturally adapted eating patterns while living in the modern world.

——— ◆ ———

Natural Eating is the art, under modern conditions, of getting close to our naturally adapted eating patterns.

——— ◆ ———

Chapter Four

What is Going Wrong

The Human Food Acquisition Apparatus

This seemingly pompous term is nevertheless good shorthand to describe the business of getting food from the environment and turning it into something used by the body.

It means collecting the food out of the environment, getting it to the mouth, the passage from the mouth through the digestive system, the transit from the digestive system into the bloodstream, and finally metabolization in the body cells into something useful.

Various types of creatures have evolved different patterns of doing this. They feed on different types of food, so their body design for *collection* is specialized. Thus the eagle has his curved beak and talons, and the hummingbird has his needle shaped beak.

The type of food decides the type of mouth, jaws and teeth. The type of food goes on to decide the configuration of the digestive system, the digestive processes (the enzymes and digestive agents) and the type of body biochemistry.

We can understand a lot about the naturally adapted human feeding pattern by seeing how it fits with what we know about other creatures.

Contrary to popular misconception, human beings are not 'omnivores' meaning capable of eating anything. Indeed it is virtually impossible to design a digestive system that could cope with the contradictory requirements of true omnivory and no example exists in nature.

Nevertheless, today people eat as though they are omnivores! So it is not surprising that diet-induced illness and poor digestion are so prevalent.

A study of the human-like 'hominoid' great apes, the gorilla, chimpanzee, orangutan, and the gibbon all show that their diets are largely vegetarian, supplemented to a greater or lesser degree by animal matter.

Gorillas concentrate mostly on leafy material and bark as does, to a lesser extent, the orangutan. Chimpanzees favor fruits more and some foliage with perhaps some 10% animal matter.

Surprisingly, it is difficult to be precise about the true dimensions of a digestive system. The various parts of the system are particularly elastic and the proportions can vary significantly from one individual to another.

According to individual dietary practices, the stomach can be small or distended, the colon longer or shorter. Indeed, a baby's colon has proportions similar to those of other apes. As humans mature, their colon, relatively speaking, shortens. But this may only happen to Westerners on a low fibre diet. We don't know enough about that yet. Nevertheless it is suggestive that in other apes the opposite happens – their colons get longer with age. It would be surprising if ours were not intended to do the same.

Of course most measurements are done on corpses (both human and ape). This presents a further difficulty, since in death, these very elastic tissues contract to the point where it is difficult to estimate their dimensions when alive.

We can make some judgements about the components that make up a digestive system. All hominoids, including humans, share the same basic pattern. They have a simple stomach, a modest-sized cecum, and a pouched or corrugated colon.

Hominoids also have an appendix. This is an unusual structure and contrary to popular belief, it serves a useful purpose. It secretes digestive agents such as mucin, eripsin and amylase, and is a powerful producer of anti-bodies for the immune system. The only other creatures that have an appendix are folivores like the rabbit and the capybara[1].

Our jaws are designed to bite out of a fruit which has been brought up to our mouths by a hand admirably designed for the purpose. Our jaws and molars are designed for masticating and grinding. Like the great apes, we have front teeth in the shape of a spade – good for biting the end off a carrot. Our saliva contains an enzyme, ptyalin, for the pre-digestion of carbohydrates (both good and bad), the predominant component of fruit and vegetation.

Chimpanzees and baboons use their hands a great deal to prepare their food. It is no coincidence that the same hand, with its ability to grasp an object, is also one that is good for grasping a branch. Like us, these creatures show great dexterity picking out the choice part of a plant or unwrapping a leaf to find a grub inside.

Finally, some more circumstantial evidence. Humans are one of the few mammals to have ball joints in the shoulder and hip. Other mammals have simple hinges. Why ball joints? They are 'universal' joints, having all degrees of movement. Why is this useful? After all, it makes the golf swing more unreliable! The only other creatures that have this facility are ones

---

1 The capybara is a large, vegetarian South American semi-aquatic creature related to the cavy and the guinea pig.

that live in trees – the primates including the chimpanzee and the gorilla. Ball joints in the limbs are essential for the gymnastics of swinging through the branches of the forest canopy. And they feed on what they find in trees.

Are Humans Carnivores?

Pure carnivores, such as cats and dogs, do not have a digestive system proportioned like a human's. They have a much larger stomach or a large stomach *and* a voluminous small intestine. In comparison, they have only a rudimentary cecum and colon.

Humans who eat a lot of meat and very little vegetation do not give their colon any work to do. It just becomes a sewer which loses tone. If you don't use it you lose it! The gut becomes prey to constipation, bowel cancers and diverticulosis.

Carnivores have long muzzles and sharp, widely spaced teeth suitable for biting and tearing into living flesh. Carnivores do not need a toothpick after a meat meal like humans do. They do not have molars for grinding (like we do). More surprisingly, their jaws cannot even move sideways in a grinding motion like ours can. Detailed study of the design of the teeth and enamel of carnivores show strong differences from those of humans and the great apes. Our teeth are excellently designed for the comminution of leafy and fruit-like material.

Furthermore, humans do not have muzzles, their faces are flat. And human fingernails are barely suitable for tearing the skin off a rice pudding!

Most mammal carnivores also have incredibly powerful jaw muscles. Hyenas and lions can readily crack open thigh bones. Humans, in comparison, have weak jaw muscles – hardly strong enough to shell a peanut!

> Humans are not designed as carnivores.

A word about 'design'.

The word 'design' is used a great deal in this book. Its meaning is intended to be in the restricted sense of a 'pattern'. There is no intention to imply or deny that a 'design' suggests the presence of a 'designer'.

A special word about eggs, insects and small creatures:

Human biochemistry seems to deal quite well with eggs – the much bruited dangers of their cholesterol content not posing a health problem in reality. There is no doubt that our Pleistocene ancestors ate eggs when they could get hold of them. There would have been seasonal periods of availability, then nothing for a while. Curiously, eggs (along with most animal proteins) are more readily digested raw which is just how they would have been eaten at the time.

A supermarket egg differs from those found in the African savannah as it comes from a chicken, a bird unknown in those parts. Even so, in order to be viable, an egg of any kind has to fit into quite a tight specification. It is at the margins that the difference is noticed. A bird that ranges and browses freely produces eggs that, inter alia, have a much better fatty acid profile than the average supermarket hen's egg. A hen that scratches in the farmyard, produces an egg that is far healthier both for its chick and for humans.

It is also true that the human digestive apparatus and biochemistry cope fine with modest quantities of insects, bugs, caterpillars, shellfish, frogs and the like. These were all available to the "human food acquisition apparatus." Some creatures, but not humans, secrete special enzymes (e.g. chitinase) to digest the hard covering (chitin) of insects. Our ancestors certainly extracted the meat from the inside and threw away the shell.

The main point remains that a digestive system can be designed for digestion of predominantly vegetation, predominantly meat, or predominantly fruit. It can even be designed to combine these possibilities two at a time, either a fruit/meat diet (as with certain New World monkeys, lemurs and lorises), a vegetation/meat diet (unknown amongst primates) or a vegetation/fruit diet (very common to primates, including the great apes, gibbons, New and Old World monkeys), but not a diet where all three have equal weight. The requirements are incompatible. Note too, the difficulties of combining just the two elements, fruit and meat *simultaneously*. (Chapter Five, *How and What We Eat*). In the wild, consumption of these different food groups toggles between either one or the other according to availability, so this risk is largely averted.

Humans are designed for a predominantly vegetation/fruit diet with animal matter an essential component in secondary position.

Are Humans Ruminants (grass eaters)?

Ruminants, such as cattle and sheep, have several stomachs and symbiotic bacteria in order to digest vast quantities of high cellulose matter like grasses. Humans do not have several stomachs with grass digesting bacteria. Sadly, this has often been put to the test in case of famine. Starving people, like in the famines of medieval Europe and Victorian Ireland, resorted to eating grass. Their mouths would be green from their 'grazing', but it did not save them. Humans are a couple of stomachs short.

> Humans are not designed as ruminants.

Are Humans Granivores (grain eaters)?

Grain eaters, such as chickens, have 'crops' and swallow stones to mill the seed which they have swallowed. Humans do not have crops and do not swallow stones. Grain eaters have special enzymes for the digestion of raw flour. They have guts that are devoted to the digestion of starch. The gut wall is full of micro-pits, and the pancreas has three ducts, one for each of the major enzyme groups.

Anyone who has tried the once fashionable 'Alpine' breakfast (where raw grains and seeds such as sesame, rye, oats and poppy are milled at the table) knows the consequences – lots of gas. Humans cannot digest raw flour. It has to be cooked or processed first.

There are other problems too. Cereals are high in phytate, a compound that interrupts the absorption of important micro-nutrients such as zinc, iron and manganese. The switch by humans to the consumption of cereals as a staple has the unintended consequence of promoting mineral deficiencies.

Fibre is an essential element in a healthy diet. But the kind of fibre makes a difference. Primates in general, and humans in particular, are good at digesting the 'dicot' vegetable fibers found in vegetation like broccoli and lettuce. These fibers are important in improving the chemical reactions that occur in the gut. Their products of digestion, once into the bloodstream, modify many vital signs such as blood lipids profiles in a healthy direction.

Primates in general are not good at digesting the 'monocot' fibers of cereal bran They are harsh on the digestive tract and, being insoluble, do not yield any useful biochemical advantage. It is interesting to note that no other Primate species attempts to eat cereals.

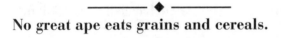

No great ape eats grains and cereals.

And what happens when, through 'processing', grains, are rendered accessible to the human digestive system? There is a sugar rush that puts enormous stress on the blood-sugar control mechanism. Human biochemistry is just not designed to cope with this phenomenon. Much more of this later.

But that is still not the end to the cereal horror. Cereals, like many other plants, have developed defenses against being eaten. These take the form of 'anti-nutrients' or toxins that are designed to upset the biochemistry of the creature that eats them. Curiously, many seed eaters (from funguses to bacteria to insects and birds) have developed resistance to these anti-nutrients. Primates, man included, have never been grain eaters and have low resistance to cereal toxins.

'Lectins' are one of the worst of these toxins. They are agglomerative

proteins with the ability to bind to carbohydrate-containing molecules anywhere in the body. They pass easily from the gut into the bloodstream and disrupt the work of any body cell that they attach themselves to. They are powerful provokers of all kinds of autoimmune disease including allergies, asthma, lupus and arthritis. They are even suspected of causing autism in susceptible children.

Worse, lectins, like the Trojan Horse, open the back door to the citadel. They cause the gut to be more porous (leaky gut syndrome) thus allowing bacteria, funguses and food particles to flood in and create their own mischief. Truly, the capacity of lectins to disrupt human health is immense.

But that is only the start of the story. There are the *alpha-amylase inhibitors.* They interrupt the activity of the starch digestion enzyme amylase and damage the pancreas. Worse, they are prominent allergens. They are at the origin of a common occupational ailment in the baking industry, "baker's asthma,' a debilitating allergic reaction to cereal flours.

Then there are the *protease inhibitors.* Cereals produce them to fight off insects and bacteria. In humans they interrupt the negative feed-back loop from the intestine which signals to the pancreas to reduce secretion. As a result the pancreas continues churning out the hormone cholecystokinin like a runaway flywheel. This disrupts normal digestive processes. More seriously, the stress on the pancreas can lead to abnormal enlargement and cancer.

Finally there are the *alkyl resorcinols.* These disrupt a wide range of body functions including disintegration of red blood cells, disruption to DNA maintenance, dramatic increase in blood-clotting and the stunting of growth.

This is an impressive catalogue of the nasty consequences of cereal poisoning.

> Humans are not designed as grain or cereal eaters.

Are Humans Lactivores (milk drinkers)?

Humans are lactivores, but only to about three years old. In common with all mammals, the new born of the species first lives off his mother's milk. *This requires a quite distinctive digestive process.* Weaning in humans, under natural conditions, happens when the child is about three years old. Until this time, the child is secreting a different set of digestive enzymes. Two important ones are *lactase* and *rennin.*

Lactase is the enzyme which helps digest *lactose* in milk. Without the enzyme, (as happens in most adults[2]), the lactose arrives in the colon

---

2 Some people, particularly of Scandinavian background, are lactase producers after weaning. But even their production of lactase diminishes with age. Frequently intolerance can suddenly develop late in life.

where it is fed upon by hydrogen-producing bacteria. Flatulence and allergic reactions can be the result.

Rennin (or rennet) is used to make cheese from milk. It is obtained from the stomachs of slaughtered unweaned calves. Cheese is therefore milk made digestible thanks to extracts from a dead calf's stomach.

Rennin is an enzyme which coagulates the milk literally into curds and whey. This is essential so that the whey, with its load of minerals, vitamins, anti-bodies and the like, can escape first into the small intestine and there get absorbed into the body. The curds, containing the proteins and fats, are held back in the stomach for digestion. Unlike an adult, the baby secretes into its stomach, a battery of protein and fat digesting enzymes.

In an adult the proteins and fats interfere with the bio-chemical metabolism of the whey. Notably, the calcium in milk is poorly absorbed. Adults, therefore, have great difficulty both in digesting milk and in extracting the goodness out of it.

What about the nature of these proteins and fats? Even they are not helpful. The proteins are dominated by casein – the protein that raises cholesterol levels the most. The fats are dominated by saturated fat and cholesterol. This is fine for babies because they are building brains. They double in size in the first six months. and brains are mostly made of fat and cholesterol. In an adult, all that fat and cholesterol is heart stopping– literally.

> Humans are not designed as milk drinkers.

A Word About Legumes[3] (lentils, garbanzo beans, beans...)

Humans do not digest pulses[3] well. With the exception of peas, most pulses contain a high percentage of indigestible oligosaccharides, notably raffinose. When they arrive in the colon, symbiotic bacteria feed on them, producing hydrogen and methane in the process. Up to 5 gallons of flatulence per day in extreme cases. Methane, particularly, is a greenhouse gas. Eating legumes contributes to global warming! Humans simply don't have the digestive enzymes necessary for the comfortable deconstruction of legumes.

Legumes are not exempt either from the same (if less potent) kinds of anti-nutrients, particularly lectins, found in cereals. Furthermore, lentils and most beans are *toxic* in the raw state. Only baking or vigorous boiling will deactivate the poison. Our prehistoric ancestors had no way to boil water, and could only bake with difficulty. We can be sure that our Pleistocene ancestors had, for the most part, less troublesome foods to eat.

With time, some creatures develop antitoxins to the toxins that are in the

3 Legumes are often called pulses and vice-versa. In this work the terms are used interchangeably.

plants that they eat. Humans developed ways of handling many toxic compounds in plant food but not for legumes. They never had to, they were not relying on legumes for food. Result, humans have neither the antitoxins nor the enzymes for the consumption of legumes. Humans are not designed as legume eaters.

This all sounds like a chamber of horrors, but we must not lose perspective. Legumes do contain much of good nutritional value, particularly proteins and many micronutrients. When put in the scale the advantages outweigh the disadvantages. If you cook them well, and can put up with the gas, legumes are a useful addition to the diet in modest portions.

———————— ◆ ————————

Although a 'novelty', legumes are a useful addition to the human diet.

———————— ◆ ————————

We can summarize the 'Human Food Acquisition Apparatus' as follows:

'Human Food Acquisition Apparatus' is good for:

- Fruit, light vegetation (salads and vegetables), nuts, some wild animal matter (including eggs)

It is not good for:

- Milk, grains and cereals, meat dominated diets, grasses and tough vegetation

---

So When Did Matters Start to Go Wrong?

The rot really set in, 10,000 years ago, when that wandering group of humans set up as farmers and *took control* of their food supply. They didn't plant what they were in the habit of eating, rather what it was *possible* to plant, harvest, store and consume.

For the first time in the history of the human race, *cereals* and *legumes* (lentils, garbanzo beans [chick peas] etc...) entered the diet in a big way. Subsequently, other foodstuffs also came into the diet for the first time.

The following timeline diagram represents how this revolution in eating habits has been accelerating right up to the present. Over the centuries, our diets have diverged ever further from our ancestral patterns, but our bodies have not changed to suit. The number of generations - about 400 - is just not enough for such changes to occur naturally. The bacteria in a human intestine go through 400 generations in a week. And we don't expect *them* to have mutated or evolved into a different creature in that time.

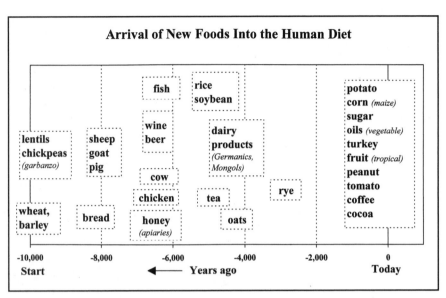

Timeline showing the arrival of new foods into the human diet

It all began about 10,000 years ago when a wandering group of humans took control of their food supply. But our bodies have not changed to suit!

What has been the result of this large and rapid change in dietary habits?

We know that:

At the introduction of cereals into the diet, the people lost stature, suffered osteo-arthritis and gum disease. Later they suffered obesity and diabetes.

With the introduction of bread, dental cavities became more prevalent.

With the introduction of domesticated animals, new diseases crossed over from the animals. Small-pox, tuberculosis, whooping cough, influenza, and measles came from the cow, the sheep, the chicken, the pig, and the dog.

With the introduction of sugar, honey, sweet corn and potato, diseases like obesity and diabetes have grown rapidly.

It is the nature of exponential change that you don't have to go back very far to find radically more primitive circumstances. So it is that the peoples of the world have, until recently, had eating habits which had not diverged greatly from those with the way our bodies are designed to function.

The Spartan foot-soldier of 2,500 years ago lived on fruit, olives, fresh figs, garden produce and rough ground barley bread. Meat was for special occasions. He had never seen sugar, maple syrup, high fructose corn syrup, maltose, sweet corn, potatoes, pasta or polished rice. Honey was an expensive luxury.

The situation changed gradually until the industrial revolution hit Europe and North America in the 19th century. Since that time there has been a sea-change in our eating habits. And since the Second World War the change has grown geometrically.

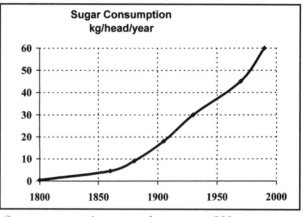

Sugar consumption was almost zero 200 years ago. Consumption has increased exponentially since then.

As an example, this chart shows how dramatically our consumption of sugar has soared.

Indeed, one major health indicator, obesity, has been rising exponentially in America and England. Both peoples are getting porkier at a frightening rate – in spite of the success in reducing dietary fat.

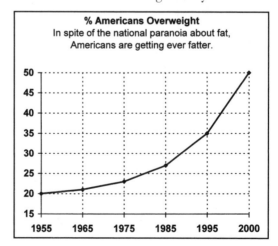

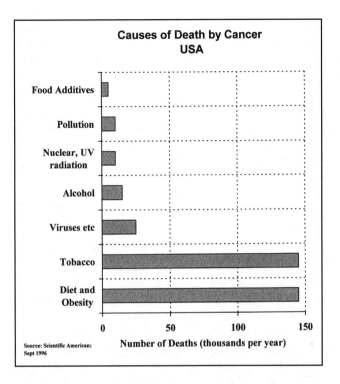

From the above chart it can be seen that most deaths by cancer (300,000 per year) are caused by our own bad habits. All other causes pale into insignificance. We can stop smoking and we can get our diet and obesity under control. In other words, we can decide whether or not to die of cancer. On the whole, Americans have not so decided. Witness this graph of cancer mortality in the US.

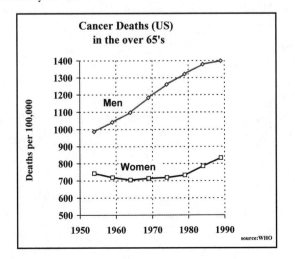

There is even a tendency to complacency. After all, hasn't human life been described as "mean, nasty, brutish and short?" Certainly when that was written by the philosopher Thomas Hobbes in 17th Century England, that was the sorry condition of much of the population. But it is also the sorry condition of any population which has outgrown its food supply, and the wrong sort of food to boot.

The reality is that even today our average life-spans of 70 to 80 years have not improved since Prehistoric times. This in spite of the fantastic advance of medical technology. (See "Lifespan in Historical Times" in Chapter Seven, *Top Ten Topics*)

———— ◆ ————

No Organ Should be a Weak Link

Here is an interesting concept which requires particular attention

> **Nature doesn't design creatures whose component parts wear out at different times.**

It is very simple. Evolutionary processes are constantly working to optimize design efficiency. A species whose kidneys, say, always wore out before anything else, would very rapidly evolve weaker primary organs elsewhere in the body such that they all wore out at the same time as the kidneys.

It is the same philosophy as attributed to Henry Ford. His genius, amongst many attributes, was to seek optimum design efficiency. The story is told that Ford asked his engineers one day which part of his motorcar never gave trouble. Upon being told the big-end bearing, he replied, "In that case it is over-designed! Go away and trim it down until it fails at the same time as everything else."

The same processes have silently operated to ensure that all our body-parts are designed to wear out at the same time. This opens up the tantalizing prospect that, if we can avoid wrecking any particular body organ, then the body as a whole just has to keep going.

This is what happens with today's centenarians. By a combination of luck and good management, they have optimized the body's ageing process. Centenarians have achieved by chance the life expectancy that is everyone's heritage.

———— ◆ ————

Today's centenarians achieve the heritage that is everyone's due.

———— ◆ ————

So the challenge today is to avoid wrecking body parts. Not only is it wasteful of life, it is very unpleasant dying prematurely with diseased and corrupted organs. A massive techno/medical industry, consuming a vast treasure – 13% of GDP in the USA – is deployed to patch up bodies that have become decrepit and prey to all kinds of degenerative disease.

Just returning to the eating patterns of our Pleistocene ancestors should ensure that we lead healthy, athletic lives, in good shape to the end. Just think how well we could do if we added the positive aspects of medical technology as well.

————— ◆ —————

Our Body's Incredibly Complex Chemical Factory

and the Sorcerer's Apprentice Syndrome

Today it is realized that the bio-chemical processes that maintain our bodies are much more complex than anyone ever realized. In just one tiny cell (quite invisible to the naked eye) a plan of all the chemical interactions would look like a three dimensional television circuit diagram, only thousands of times more complex. A veil is lifted on just one tiny corner in the Sample Hormone Cascade further on in this chapter. Further, our bodies contain some 50 trillion cells, all churning away like miniature chemical factories.

There are two important things to realize. The pathways form a *network*, and the ramifications are fiendishly complicated. By meddling in this process we are like the sorcerer's apprentice who only knows a part of the story.

By trying to do good he only made things worse. This is often how we are when we take supplements, medications and unhelpful foods.

And the point about the network is that a change in one compound has knock-on effects in unexpected directions. Alternatively, if one route is blocked, then there are *alternative paths* to the same objective.

How are we to micromanage this? The answer is, *we don't*. Our own bodies are perfectly adapted to managing these processes all by themselves. But we have to send clear messages, and we have to give our bodies the tools to do the job.

When we eat badly – eat in ways that are discordant with the blueprint – that scrambles the body's micromanagement. When we eat the Western diet we are like a bull in a china shop. Every move is breaking the china.

There are many manifestations of so-called food/disease connections. One of the less familiar is the food/arthritis connection. This is a disease that is becoming widespread under the influence of poor dietary practices. One of these is the aberrant consumption of essential fatty acids. Remember these from Chapter Three?

Today, the American diet is hopelessly overbalanced in favor of linoleic acid, typically corn oil, sunflower oil, peanut oil and the like. Linoleic acid is converted into a series of different hormones that can be either *beneficial or harmful*. What decides the way it goes? Other dietary practices.

This sample hormone cascade shows how linoleic acid is transformed into these hormones. See how complicated it is? The transformation is blocked if the enzyme Delta 6 Desaturase is not around. And look at what controls that. Bad carbohydrates, insulin and the like. But it gets worse. Downstream there is a switching gatekeeper, Delta 5 Desaturase. The

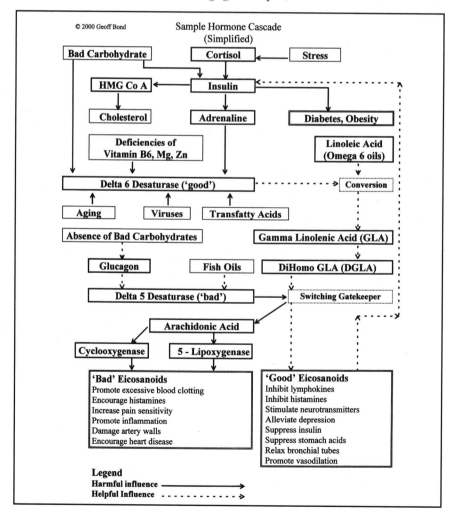

greater or lesser presence of this enzyme *decides which way* the hormonal transformation will go, into *good* or *bad* messages to the body's cells.

Some people have heard that arthritis can be helped by the consumption of GLA (Gamma Linoleic Acid). This is present in Evening Primrose Oil. But you see the catch? Of itself, taking GLA does not determine what the body is going to do with it. It could still be turned into compounds, by the Delta 5 Desaturase, that *aggravate* arthritis rather than alleviate it. It all depends what other things you are doing with your diet.

This is a classic case of 'Sorcerer's Apprentice Syndrome', meddling in half understood processes only making them worse. It is also known as the 'Law of Unintended Consequences'.

Just to make the point, look at the following diagram:

This shows the inter-relationship of various minerals, vitamins and other factors in the diet. I am not asking you to understand it. I just want you to be impressed by it.

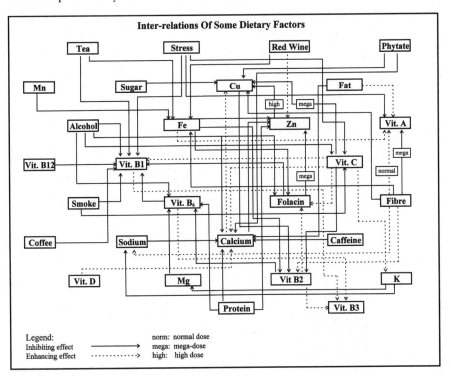

I want you to be impressed by the interdependence of all these factors. For example, consumption of calcium improves absorption of copper but depletes absorption of zinc. Or, consumption of red wine helps zinc absorption but inhibits iron absorption.

How is anyone to find the right balance? The answer is that it is impossible.

As ever, the answer is to consume our foods in the right proportions, in the proportions for which the body is naturally adapted. The body will do the rest.

Trying to compensate for dietary errors (imagined or real) by dosing up on this or that supplement only confuses other processes in unimagined ways.

The message is, it is impossible to micro-manage these processes. But then there is no need. Our own bodies are incredibly well endowed with their own self management mechanisms.

──────── ◆ ────────

Our own body is the best manager of its biochemistry.

──────── ◆ ────────

What does this mean? It means none other than to return to the pattern of eating to which our bodies have been adapted over millions of years – to that eaten by our prehistoric forebears. It is a way of eating which is in *harmony* with the way our bodies have evolved. It is *Natural*.

Chapter Five

What and How We Eat

In the previous chapters, we have been building up a case for a particular pattern of eating which is the ideal for human beings. In this chapter we look at our eating patterns today and what is right and wrong about them.

What We Eat

Here we look at the foods that have crept into the diet in the last 10,000 years and pass judgment on them. That is, judge whether they can be admitted to the 'club' and if not, if there is anything they can do to shape up.

Carbohydrates

Carbohydrates span the whole spectrum of vegetation from lettuce, broccoli and apples through to bread, cakes, and sugar.

Many carbohydrates either form a natural part of the human diet or are novelties that happen to conform to the same profile. These are termed *'favorable'* carbohydrates.

Others are marginal foods. Either they are novelties that don't quite make the grade, or they are modern adaptations that have become marginal. These are termed *'borderline'* carbohydrates.

Finally, there is a category of *'bad'* carbohydrates. These are foods that humans were never designed to consume. Typically they are sugars, cereals and other starches.

How are the categories decided upon? The worst characteristic that a carbohydrate can have is to be *highly glycemic.* This is its power to raise blood sugar levels to dangerous levels.

One of the most dangerous dietary errors committed today is the consumption of bad carbohydrates on a massive scale. The result is *blood sugar levels* out of control. Why does this happen?

The human body chemistry is designed to work with a low octane fuel – plant food. It cannot cope with large quantities of 'rocket fuel', notably simple sugars and bad starches.

Simple sugars and bad starches are quickly converted to glucose, which rapidly enters the bloodstream. The bloodstream has to maintain blood

---

Typical Favorable Carbohydrates:

lettuce, tomatoes, cherries, apples, broccoli, grapefruit, mushroom.
See Appendix 1, Table 5 for more.

Typical Borderline Carbohydrates:

ripe banana, rice, oatmeal, dried fruits, macaroni.
See Appendix 1, Table 4 for more.

glucose levels within close limits. This is done by the pancreas[1] releasing the hormone *insulin* into the bloodstream. The quantities of insulin are dosed in accordance with the arrival of glucose. If the arrival of glucose is rapid, the pancreas cannot maintain this orderly matching of insulin to glucose. Initially, the pancreas does not react fast enough and there is an *overdose* of glucose in the bloodstream. This condition is known as *hyperglycemia*. An excess of glucose in the blood kills nerve endings and damages blood vessels.

Kidney disease, blindness and amputations are the consequence of chronic hyperglycemia.

Then the pancreas catches up and *overcompensates*. A sudden excess peak of glucose in the bloodstream is mopped up by a flash flood of insulin which is in excess of that needed. There is now a *deficiency* of glucose in the blood. This condition is known as *hypoglycemia*. It is characterized by feelings of drowsiness, dizziness, irritability, exhaustion, cold sweats, depression, headaches, etc. These feelings are accompanied by a desperate craving for something sugary.

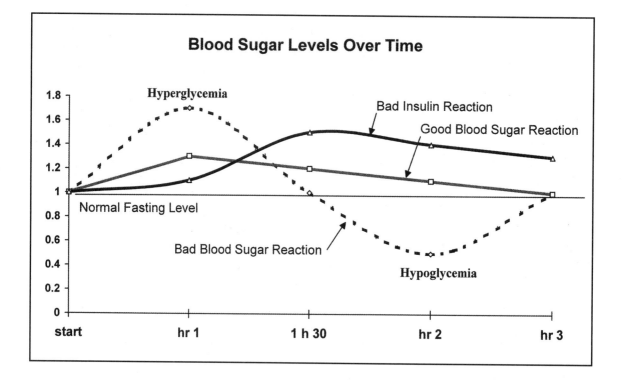

1 The pancreas is a multifunction organ that secretes a wide variety of hormones and digestive enzymes under instruction from other parts of the body.

The chart on page 74 shows:

- a normal glucose reaction, where the rising level of glucose in the blood is carefully mastered and brought under control. There is no abnormal peak of glucose. The glucose level never drops below the normal fasting level.

- a bad reaction, where the glucose concentration rises to an abnormally high level (hyperglycemia). Later the glucose concentration drops below the normal fasting level. (hypoglycemia).

But worse, this switchback of blood sugar levels results in a cascade of debilitating diseases: diabetes, heart disease, blocked arteries, kidney disease, obesity and various immune system disorders such as cancer, arthritis and allergies.

How does this come about? High blood sugar levels mean high insulin levels. This is a biochemical disaster. Insulin is a powerful hormone. One of its functions is to cause the cells to sweep up excess glucose out of the blood and so bring the glucose concentration back to normal. But at the same time it is also sweeping fat into the fat cells.

The story gets worse. Insulin floating around in abnormal quantities (known as 'hyperinsulinemia') upsets all other kinds of hormonal reactions. Remember those diagrams in Chapter Four? Most people who have high cholesterol levels have it *because their body is making it.* The insulin effectively instructs the liver to make more than necessary. Similar mechanisms increase blood clotting, damage arteries, suppress the immune system (allowing cancers to grow), even cause the bones to lose calcium.

The problem with hyperinsulinemia is that you don't even feel it! You cannot feel if your insulin levels are out of control. Hyperinsulinemia goes about its work silently, you notice nothing until it is too late and you have the stroke, the heart attack, the cancer is expressed, your bones are like Swiss cheese, your arteries are sludged up.

Think of the phenomenon like the iceberg that sank the Titanic. You see very little on the surface, but underneath lurks mortal danger. You just see some disconnected peaks, but under the surface they are all linked.

So how do we avoid 'abnormal' blood sugar levels? Very simply by not consuming foodstuffs which contain bad carbohydrates. You can start today and you will start to feel the benefits straight away. If you are already hyperglycemic then be prepared. At several places throughout the book, food is talked about as a kind of drug. This is where the truth of that statement will be borne in on you. Just like any junky going cold turkey you will get withdrawal symptoms such as cold sweats, headaches, and a craving for the drug that you are trying to abandon, sugar in all its forms.

> Diabetes is a common result of bad carbohydrate abuse. The pancreas fails, or the fat cells become insensitive.

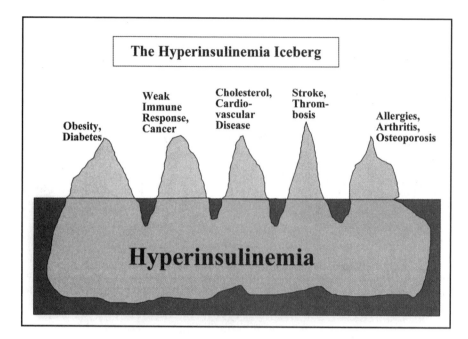

How do we know what *bad* carbohydrates are? A new tool has been developed recently which gives guidance. It is known as the *Glycemic Index.*

Glycemic Index and Peak Blood Sugar Levels

The glycemic index is a measure of the sugar rush that a carbohydrate dumps into the bloodstream. The higher the index, the worse for you. Originally the index was set at 100 for glucose itself, but later it was discovered that maltose (as found in beer) is even higher. (This explains the mechanism by which beer drinkers are more likely to develop a 'beer belly' whereas wine drinkers are less likely to.)

It has to be understood that the measurement of glycemic index is not a terribly precise science. According to the variability of the food and the variability of the feeder, the glycemic index can vary. However it is precise enough to tell us all that we need to know. It tells us enough to confirm or deny our worst fears, and help us to choose wisely. (see Appendix 1, Glycemic Indexes)

Broadly, carbohydrates are classified by glycemic index as shown in this table. The divisions between the categories is necessarily arbitrary, but it is a good rule of thumb.

Carbohydrate Class	Range of G.I.
bad	65 and above
borderline	35 to 65
favorable	zero to 35

How are we to know the glycemic index, unless we are told it? The answer is, we don't. The only way to know the G.I. for a particular food is to feed it to volunteers under controlled conditions and then measure their blood sugar level at half-hour intervals.

When this was first done in the early 1980's it revolutionized the way carbohydrates were viewed. The researchers were astonished to find that the 'common sense' medical advice to prefer 'complex carbohydrates[2]' was misguided. It turned out that wholewheat bread was no better than white bread, which in turn was no better than sugar itself. Or, that the cornflake itself was just as bad as the honey coating.

The only 'safe' foods (surprise, surprise) were the 'very complex carbohydrates[2]' such as green and yellow leafy vegetables and low sucrose fruits. In other words, human beings have a biochemistry perfectly adapted to this kind of carbohydrate. That is how our bodies are made, and that is the kind of fuel to give them.

Human beings' biochemistry is over-stressed by sugars, starchy carbohydrates (as found in cereals and grains) and some tubers (like potatoes). These are substances that have intruded into the human diet very recently. They have major drawbacks and we have no business consuming them.

Since the time of the first researches, hundreds of carbohydrates have been studied and their glycemic indexes evaluated. A short selection is given in Appendix 1, Tables 3-5. A full list is published in the Natural Eating Manual.

If the food you want is not in any of the tables? You can make a reasonable assessment by finding analogies with similar foods. But the real question is what are you doing eating a food about which you have doubts anyway?

If the food has an ingredient label, that very fact means that it is processed and is a confection of many additives and ingredients. Its effect on the body biochemistry is unknowable and therefore such a food is suspect.

Food labels need to get a lot more sophisticated before the consumer will have all the information to make wise choices. In Europe for example, there is a brand of very dark, low sugar chocolate that mentions its glycemic index on the packet. It has a low G.I. of just 22. What do you know – a safe confectionery item!

A move to labeling like this would be a tremendous help, not only to consumers, but also in creating a more frank mentality amongst manufacturers about their products.

---

2 Carbohydrates had originally been classified into 'simple' and 'complex'. The simple carbohydrates are sugars whose molecules are simple in structure and were consequently thought to be rapidly absorbed. The complex carbohydrates are chiefly starches whose molecule is complicated and were consequently thought to take longer to absorb. This assumption ignored the remarkable power of digestive enzymes to speed up chemical processes thousands of times. In reality, bread hits the bloodstream as soon as sugar does. A new category of carbohydrates has been gaining currency, the 'very complex carbohydrates'. These are the colored plant foods rich in various oligosaccharides that are both complex and slower to digest.

That is a tour around the concept of glycemic index (G.I.). *Refer to the tables in Appendix 1 regularly* until their contents are completely familiar to you. Try to get a feel for which kind of foodstuff falls into which category. That way, you will negotiate your way with confidence through the minefield of dubious products offered for consumption today. Take your reading glasses when you go shopping and READ THE SMALL PRINT!

Make a conscious effort to ditch the bad carbohydrates. Make a conscious effort to concentrate your meals on the favorable carbohydrates. Be cautious with the borderline carbohydrates. Paying serious attention to this question is one of the most important steps in restructuring your eating habits.

The question of G.I. has been treated at some length in this section on carbohydrates. It just remains to mention one other criterion for classifying carbohydrates.

The carbohydrates that humans are designed to eat are high micro-nutrient density and high in soluble fibers. Classically, they are represented by fruit, vegetation (salads and vegetables), tubers, nuts and berries. Many other carbohydrates are micro-nutrient poor (such as sugars and cereals) and even protein poor (such as yams, cassava and Indian corn). It so happens that, with very few exceptions, they are also the foodstuffs that are highly glycemic.

A composite table of 'Good Foods To Eat In Bulk' is presented in Appendix 1 Table 1, and of 'Good Foods to be Eaten in Controlled Quantities' in Appendix 1, Table 2.

The Bottom Line on Carbohydrates

Eat unrestricted *Favorable* carbohydrates COPIOUSLY.

AVOID *Bad* Carbohydrates.

Proteins

The human race is adapted to get its proteins as much from vegetation as animal matter.

One of the greatest errors committed today is the over-consumption of protein in general and of animal protein in particular. It is estimated that on average Americans consume double the recommended daily amount of protein from all sources. This leads to negative calcium balance and osteoporosis, kidney disease, detoxification overload, acidosis and various digestive disorders.

The modest quantities of meat consumed by the human race in its evolutionary history were quite different in nature from what is available today. The problem with 'farm' meat is that it has been bred over millennia for high fat content. As bad luck would have it, the fat is highly saturated and it doesn't even have the saving grace of containing essential fatty acids (vitamin F).

Wild game meat has a much lower fat content (4%) and contains a good percentage of EFA's. Yet this form of meat is inaccessible to the vast majority of the Western population.

A good compromise is skinless chicken and turkey breast. They are only 4% fat, albeit not the best fatty acid profile.

There is more leeway than we are led to believe in the body's need for protein. For example, it has remarkable powers to compensate for low protein intake by resorbing and recycling waste proteins in the gut. Curiously, the total amount of protein consumed is less important than the amount of starch consumed with it. A high starch/protein ratio is more likely to lead to protein deficiency than lack of protein itself.

The only peoples in the world who suffer protein deficiency are those whose staple diet is based on high starch/protein ratio, protein-impoverished starches such as cassava[3] and Indian corn. Only worry about protein deficiency if you base your diet on empty calories (e.g. popcorn, hominy, sugar and alcohol).

Our consumption of protein needs to fall between quite close limits – neither too little, nor too much. How do you manage this? You know the answer. Get your eating pattern right and the quantities work out just right.

> **The Bottom Line on Proteins**
>
> Eat naturally
> and the protein quantity works out just right

> Many people have doubts about consuming animal flesh.
>
> As set out in the introduction, we leave such ethical considerations to the judgement of the individual reader

Fats and Oils

The Human race is designed for a very low fat diet.

The only fats that the body needs are the essential fatty acids, linoleic and alpha linolenic acid. (vitamins F_1 & F_2) They are *polyunsaturated* fats and they need to be consumed in the ratio of between 4 and 1:1. This is how they occur in nature, present in about every form of vegetation.

The great dietary errors committed today are three-fold:

• too much fat and oil is consumed

3 Cassava, also called manioc, is an edible tuber from the American tropics probably first cultivated by the Maya. Its flour, bread and tapioca are widely consumed throughout the tropics. People who rely too much on it develop the deficiency disease kwashiorkor.

• the fats and oils are the wrong kind

• the EFA ratio is hopelessly unbalanced

It is unrealistic to think that in today's world oils and fats are not going to be used. The defensive strategy is to keep them to a minimum and to ensure that they have the right nutritive profile.

There are two great disasters that have overtaken the Western consumer in the last fifty years. The first is well known: the increase in consumption of saturated fat. This comes from two main sources, increased consumption of farm meat, and increased consumption of dairy products. Both of these are intruders in the human diet and carry with them a strong potential for undermining health. The problem with saturated fat is its potential to drive a coach and horses through the essential fatty acid hormonal cascade. (Remember the diagram in Chapter Four?). Saturated fat also depresses the immune system and other vital metabolic processes.

The second disaster is less well known. It is the dramatic increase in the consumption of vegetable oils, notably the so-called 'Omega 6' oils. These are oils like sunflower oil, corn oil, peanut oil and safflower oil. Virtually unknown until World War II they now take a major share of the increased fat consumption. What is the problem with Omega 6 oils? They are too cheap and easily available! Hence the over-consumption.

More seriously, these vegetable oils totally monopolize the Fatty Acid Hormonal Cascade (diagram in Chapter Four). They crowd out the alpha-linolenic acid pathway and lead to the over-production of certain hormones, which then harm health.

The following diagram portrays how this happens. If you imagine the

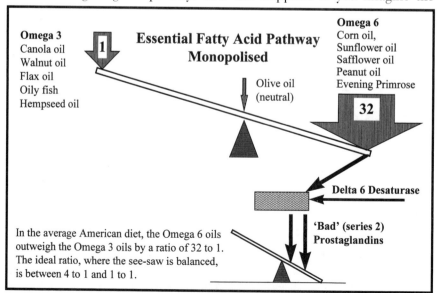

Omega 3
Canola oil
Walnut oil
Flax oil
Oily fish
Hempseed oil

1

Essential Fatty Acid Pathway Monopolised

Olive oil
(neutral)

Omega 6
Corn oil,
Sunflower oil
Safflower oil
Peanut oil
Evening Primrose

32

Delta 6 Desaturase

In the average American diet, the Omega 6 oils outweigh the Omega 3 oils by a ratio of 32 to 1. The ideal ratio, where the see-saw is balanced, is between 4 to 1 and 1 to 1.

'Bad' (series 2) Prostaglandins

competing pathways as being on opposite sides of a see-saw, then the overweight Omega 6 playground bully holds his end down leaving the Omega 3 lightweight helplessly kicking his legs in the air!

This in turn leads to the over production of 'bad' hormones. These are responsible for the roll call of bad effects listed in the box.

Truly, humans have no business consuming bulk[4] vegetable oils!

There is only one bulk oil which really complies with the ideal profile: canola oil, also known as colza oil or rapeseed oil. It is also possible to find 'spreads' made from it.

Other oils which are fine are walnut oil and flaxseed (linseed) oil. Hempseed oil, so far only available in Europe, has an excellent profile. Olive oil's main quality is that it is not Omega 6 or saturated. Its influence on the body's metabolism is neutral.

'Bad' Prostaglandins encourage:

- *plaque formation (sclerosis)*
- *immune depression (cancer)*
- *blood clotting (thromboses)*
- *inflammation (arthritis)*
- *histamines (allergies)*
- *vasoconstriction (blood pressure)*
- *hypertension (high blood pressure)*
- *auto-immune reactions (arthritis)*
- *insulin overproduction*
- *bronchial constriction (asthma)*
- *neurotransmitter suppression (pain)*

This diagram shows the ideal balance of essential fatty acids for good health.

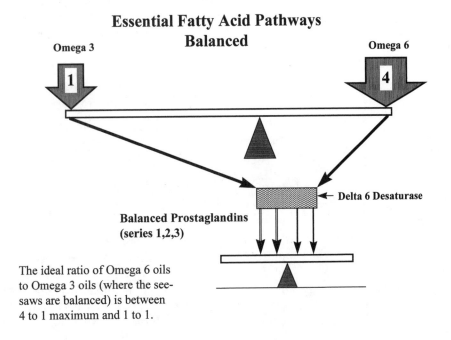

Essential Fatty Acid Pathways
Balanced

Omega 3 **1** Omega 6 **4**

← Delta 6 Desaturase

Balanced Prostaglandins (series 1,2,3)

The ideal ratio of Omega 6 oils to Omega 3 oils (where the see-saws are balanced) is between 4 to 1 maximum and 1 to 1.

---

4 In nature oils never occur on their own, they always come associated with proteins (as in fish and nuts) carbohydrates (as in corn and sunflower) or both. It is most unnatural for oils to be available in bulk and our bodies are not designed to cope with that.

All fats are suspect. Their solid nature betrays the presence of large quantities of saturated fats. Also avoid *trans-fatty acid* and *hydrogenated fats*. They are just as bad as saturated fats. These all have the effect of sabotaging the Hormonal Cascade altogether. If you eat too much saturated, hydrogenated and transfatty acids, it doesn't matter how much of the essential fatty acids you consume, their metabolization will be blocked, and you will suffer vitamin F (EFA) deficiency.

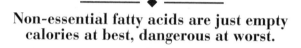

Saturated fats provoke vitamin F deficiency.

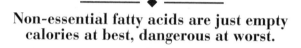

Fatty Acids Under the Microscope

We have talked a great deal about essential fatty acids (vitamins F_1 and F_2). They are part of the *polyunsaturated* fatty acid series. All you need to hold onto is that all other fatty acids are just empty calories at best and quite harmful at worst.

Non-essential fatty acids are just empty calories at best, dangerous at worst.

What are the non-essential fatty acids? We have all heard of the bogeymen – *saturated fats*. It is less commonly known that they form a series. The main ones present in food are *lauric acid, stearic acid, myristic acid* and *palmitic acid*. In reality, they have different degrees of 'badness'.

And then, of course, there are the 'goody' *monounsaturated* fatty acids like *oleic acid* as found in olive oil. Having read this far, you will appreciate that their 'goodness' resides mostly in the fact that they do no harm – they are still chiefly empty calories.

Just know that it is possible to steer your way through the minefield of modern foodstuffs guided by the curiosities of fatty acid chemistry. There is not space in this book to go into all the subtleties (for this refer to the Natural Eating Manual). Here is an overview to give you a taste of the possibilities.

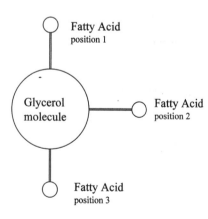

Triglyceride Molecule

Fatty acids are present in our food and in our bloodstream mostly as *triglycerides*. A triglyceride is a molecule of glycerol to which three fatty acids are attached – in positions 1, 2 and 3. (see the diagram) Now comes a clever part. When we eat a triglyceride, it is split down into its component parts in the digestive tract and then it gets reconstructed as a different triglyceride in the bloodstream.

Now comes a second clever part. Depending on the fatty acid's position (1, 2 or 3) on the molecule, so it is more or less bio-available. Thus, in reality cocoa butter is much less cholesterolemic than in theory because its saturated fatty acids are in positions 1 and 3. The digestive system is less efficient at deconstructing fatty acids in these positions and as a result they are less likely to be absorbed into the body. This effect is accentuated when calcium salts are formed. This appears to be the explanation for the relatively harmless effect of cheese fats.

All this might seem complicated – and it is! Indeed, it is so complicated that the full picture is still being worked out. Once again, you do not have to try to micromanage these processes. But you should understand that this is why it is possible to admit some, on the face of it unpromising, fatty foodstuffs (like avocado and cocoa butter) into the Natural Eating Pattern. It is also why others, like coconut (meat, oil, milk and butter) should be used with caution.

The Bottom Line on Fats and Oils

- Eat as little oil and fat as possible.
- What you do eat should be rich in both essential fatty acids.
- The best oils are canola (best, and good for most uses), walnut oil (e.g. use as condiment) and flaxseed oil (e.g. use as condiment).
- You can also include an 'oily' fish a few times a week (optional).
- Banish 'bad' fats and oils.

Note that olive oil is neither good nor bad, and it is still empty calories.

Dairy Products

The Human race is not designed for the consumption of dairy products. (See Chapter Four.)

Milk is strictly for unweaned babies. Only babies are supplied with the enzymes (rennet, lactase etc.) for the proper digestion and treatment of milk.

Adults who drink milk run the risk of protein over-consumption and osteoporosis, indigestion and flatulence, allergies, and clogged arteries from the saturated fat.

Anyone who eats butter and cream is increasing risk of heart disease, clogged arteries and all the ills attributed to blocked metabolism of essential fatty acids. (See the horror story in the previous section.)

Cheese, although an artifact of man's ingenuity, is probably tolerable in small quantities. Its saturated fat would appear to be poorly absorbed, and the lactose problem has been more or less eliminated in the manufacturing process. However the cholesterol-raising casein (a protein) content is a concern.

Yogurt again is a man-made artifact. The low fat variety is probably tolerable in small quantities. The protein content is still the cholesterol raising sort, but the lactose problem has been overcome in the fermentation process.

The Bottom Line on Dairy Products

You will be healthier if you never eat a dairy product again in your life

• Milk is definitely not recommended.

• Butter is definitely harmful.

• Cream is definitely harmful.

But:

• Low fat yogurt is tolerated in frugal quantities.

• Cheese is tolerated in frugal quantities.

Welcome Migrants to the Human Diet

In Chapter Four we had a look at all the 'novelty' foods that came into the human diet since the farming revolution 10,000 years ago. In this chapter we have so far frightened ourselves by examining the harm that many of them do to our health. Now let's give ourselves some encouragement. Let us grant a passport into our kitchen to favorable 'novelty' foods.

Here is a selection of the most common together with their pros and cons.

Legumes:

The welcome mat was already rolled out in Chapter Four. As a reminder:

Legumes are a fine source of vegetable protein.

Legumes are a good source of calories.

Legumes, particularly soy bean, contain useful micro-nutrients.

But:

Legumes are more or less toxic. They must be well cooked.

Legumes cause flatulence in many people.

Legumes contain varying amounts of anti-nutrients such as lectins.

Tomatoes

The tomato belongs to the nightshade family of plants and is closely related to bell-peppers, potato, tobacco and deadly nightshade (belladonna). Most nightshades, including the potato, but excluding the tomato, contain poisonous alkaloids. The alkaloids are destroyed on cooking.

The tomato was brought to Europe in the 16th Century by the Spanish conquistadors who found it with the Incas in Peru. It took another three centuries before it was bred into its modern forms and accepted into the food supply. Since the 19th Century, the tomato has become an integral part of many cuisines.

Tomatoes are packed with valuable health helpful micro-nutrients.

Tomatoes are flavorful, cheap and readily available.

Tomatoes, even in processed form (canned, paste, ketchup), still retain much of their nutritional value.

Tomatoes can be eaten either as a fruit or a vegetable.

But:

Tomatoes are strongly acidic[5] and, in susceptible people, can give digestive difficulties either on their own or in combination with other foods, particularly starches.

Tea

Tea is a native of the area bounded by Tibet, Northern India and China. It was first cultivated and drunk as a beverage some 5,000 years ago. Both green tea and black tea come from the same type of plant, just the drying and fermenting are slightly different.

Tea contains powerful anti-oxidants and other micro-nutrients which are helpful to health.

Tea is cheap, flavorful and freely available.

Tea, due to its mild caffeine content, has an agreeably stimulating property.

But:

Tea contains 'anti-nutrients' such as tannins, that can inactivate micro-

---

5 Tomatoes are acid to the taste and to the digestive system but, once metabolized, have an alkalizing effect on body fluids. See the segment later in this chapter, The Acid/Alkali Balance in the Body.

nutrients ingested at the same time.

Tea contains a mild dose of caffeine. In moderation this is acceptable. (See Chapter Seven). Decaffeinated tea is fine.

Coffee

Coffee originated in Ethiopia and has been used by the Arabic cultures for many centuries. It only appeared in the West during the 17th Century.

Coffee is flavorful and readily available.

Modest consumption of weak (American) coffee has no adverse effects.

Coffee, due to its caffeine content, has agreeable stimulating properties.

Coffee contains micro-nutrients that are helpful to health.

But:

Coffee contains strong concentrations of caffeine that if taken in excess can have detrimental effects on health. Decaffeinated coffee is fine.

Dry Wine (Red and White)

Pots were fabricated for the first time about 8,000 years ago in the Near East. Within a few years wine had been invented! In ancient times wine was much drunk, but diluted with water – it seems that otherwise the taste wasn't too great.

Wine today is a flavorful and agreeable beverage.

Wine in moderation, through its modest alcohol content, has a pleasant relaxing effect.

Wine contains anti-oxidants and other micro-nutrients that are health helpful.

But:

Wine in excess is health harmful.

Chicken Breast, Turkey Breast

Chicken was first domesticated about 6,000 years ago in South East Asia. Turkey is much more recent; it dates from 16th Century North America.

The *skinless* breast of chicken and turkey is a low fat meat comparable to the composition of the wild game of our Pleistocene ancestors.

The *skinless* breast of chicken and turkey is a good source of animal protein

But:

The fat[6] is of borderline profile.

---

6 This is broiler chicken. Free browsing chicken will have a better fatty acid profile.

Broiler chicken has an unknown antibiotic and artificial hormone content.

Olive Oil

Olive oil has been cultivated for several thousand years. It certainly dates from biblical times.

Olive oil is a tasty, readily available oil.

Olive oil stands up well to cooking,

Olive oil is harmless to human bio-chemistry.

But:

Olive oil is empty calories.

Canola Oil

Canadian enterprises recently improved on varieties of rapeseed (colza) by removing a harmful compound, erucic acid, to produce Canola oil (whence the name).

Canola oil has an almost perfect essential fatty acid profile.

Canola oil is cheap and freely available.

But:

Even canola oil in excess of a couple of teaspoons a day is just empty calories.

Oily Fish (Salmon, Tuna, Sardine, Mackerel)

Our Pleistocene ancestors had occasional access to freshwater fish, but it is doubtful that they formed a significant part of the diet. Oily fish are typically cold, sea water fish. These fish only entered the diet in a big way since the development of ocean-going fishing industries in the 19th Century, and salmon farming in the 20th Century.

Oily fish are flavorful and readily available.

Oily fish contain very helpful oils, notably eicosapentanoic acid, a surrogate for the much sought-after alpha linolenic acid (vitamin F_2).

Cocoa

Cocoa originated in central America and only entered the diet in a big way in the 20th Century.

Cocoa makes highly appreciated confectionery.

Cocoa in its pure form is quite harmless.

Cocoa is packed with high-quality polyphenol antioxidants.

But:

Cocoa is often combined with sugar and milk in ways that make unsuitable chocolate.

The Acid/Alkali Balance in the Body

Foodstuff		Index
Very Alkaline		**BEST**
Spinach, boiled		39.6
Almonds, raw		18.3
Avocados		10.7
Celery, raw		8.4
Grapefruit		6.4
Cabbage, raw		5.6
Tomatoes, raw		5.6
Lettuce		3.8
Cucumber, raw		3.2
Apples, eating	⇧	3.0
	Alkaline	
Neutral		**ZERO**
	Acid	
Bread, toasted	⇩	-2.6
Cheese, cheddar		-5.4
Shredded wheat		-5.7
Spaghetti		-7.5
Sponge cake		-9.1
Peanuts		-11.6
Egg, fried		-16.5
Bacon, fried		-17.0
Beefsteak, grilled		-23.2
Chicken, roasted		-25.4
Very Acid		**WORST**

The over-consumption of acid-forming foods is another major dietary error today. Note that we are not talking here about foods that *taste* acid. We mean 'acid-forming' foods. These are ones that only after digestion, absorption and metabolization by the body, have the result of acidifying the body.

The products of digestion are rarely neutral. All foods will cause the blood to be either more acidic or alkaline. The body is constantly juggling to restore a neutral balance.

The average westerner is in chronic acid surplus. The body restores the balance by using an alkali to neutralize the acidity. What is this alkali? None other than one based on calcium! Consuming a relentlessly acid diet causes the body to draw down its reserves of calcium.

What are acid forming foods? They are ones that contain sulfur, phosphorus and chlorine. These elements are found chiefly in proteins like meat, fish, eggs and cheese and starches like bread, flour and cereals. For example, bland roast chicken is one of the most acidifying foods around.

What are alkali forming foods? Ones that have a predominance of metallic elements like potassium, sodium, iron and calcium. None other than fruit, salads and vegetables! Once again, the problem is not necessarily foods that taste acid. Many fruits taste acid, but by a curious bio-chemical pathway, their result in the body is *alkaline*. For example grapefruit (q.v.) although acid to the taste has a strong alkalizing effect.

Why do some acid tasting foods not acidify the body? The answer lies in what happens to the products of digestion. The acid taste of many fruits is due to the presence of organic acids such as malic acid. This acid stays intact through the mouth, through the stomach and into the intestine. At all points up to here, the effect on the digestive process and lining is acidic.

In the intestine the malic acid passes through the intestinal wall into the blood stream. Here the malic acid is broken down into smaller molecules, the net result of which is that the acid component is *exhaled* through the lungs. The acid fraction of the fruit is thus excreted, leaving the alkalizing fraction behind in the body.

The Natural Eating Pattern, not surprisingly, correctly predicts the importance of this acid/alkali balance for human beings It ensures that the ratio of acid-forming to alkali-forming foods is a healthy one of at least 75% alkali forming by weight[7].

Consuming a relentlessly acid diet causes the body to draw down its reserves of calcium.

Indexes of acidity and alkalinity have been worked out for most food-stuffs. The table on p. 88 shows the degree of acidity or alkalinity of a short, select list of foodstuffs. *(A complete list including such items as cornflakes, cabbage, popcorn and cookies, is published in the Natural Eating Manual.)*

Intestinal Health and Detoxification.

The body is endowed with a remarkable sewage treatment plant, the liver. Blood vessels carry the products of digestion to the liver. There, the liver removes most noxious substances. Where it can, it trans-forms them step by step into innocuous substances and shoots them out, with the bile, back into the beginning of the intestinal tract.

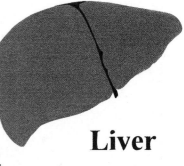

Liver

Everything is fine so long as the liver can cope with the toxic load. However all is not well with the way we eat today. Passage through the intestines is slow and consists of foods which give rise to a high level of toxic matter. In addition, this environment encourages the growth of unfriendly bacteria and fungi, which produce their own toxins.

Other foods, like hot peppers, cause the lining of the intestine to be more porous, known as 'leaky gut syndrome'. It doesn't take much. The gut wall is as thin as tissue paper. That is all that separates the gunge in your gut from the your nice clean blood circulation!

Even under good conditions, after a meal there are *always* some bacteria that pass through into the blood. For example, primitive herders (and for that matter wild west ranchers) knew to starve a beast for 24 hours before slaughter. That way there are fewer bacteria generalized throughout the carcass and the meat keeps longer.

Today, our dietary errors vastly increase both the porosity of the gut and the micro-organism load. So it is that abnormal quantities of digestion toxins, bacterial and fungal toxins, and the bacteria and fungi themselves, pass into the bloodstream. The liver cannot cope and the bacteria, fungi and toxins continue on their way to other parts of the body where they cause mischief.

They can be at the origin of various allergies, auto-immune response, or the simple poisoning of various bodily functions. All kinds of disorders can arise: headaches, arthritis, tiredness, irritability and depression.

7 Alkali forming foods, for the most part plant foods, have a high percentage of water. Most acid forming foods, the protein-rich ones, are dense. To strike the balance, the ratio of alkali forming to acid forming has to be at least 3 to 1, or 75% of the total, by weight.

Ever wondered why sometimes the contents of your bowels smell like estuary sludge? Do you ever worry about it? Well, you should! Recent research shows that this is due to the abnormal presence of sulfur-reducing bacteria. Why do they flourish? Because they feed on the sulfur-bearing amino acids in meat (sulfur again). Does it matter? Recent research has shown a link with ulcerative colitis, a serious inflammatory bowel disease. Worse, the toxic sulfides released by these bacteria promote cancerous changes in gut cells by damaging their DNA.

All this helps to explain why heavy meat eaters are more vulnerable to colon cancer. So what about vegetarians? They seem to be protected because plant proteins usually do not contain sulfur, and the protein comes in a carbohydrate package.

Finally, there is another factor, sulfur used as a preservative. Sulfur in many forms, but collectively baptized 'sulfur dioxide', is ubiquitous in the processed food industry. It is present in everything from packaged salads to jams, hamburgers, sausages, instant soup, salad bars, beer and wine. People who eat a lot of processed foods not only promote sulfur bacteria in their gut, they also raise their sensitivity to allergic reactions, and that's probably all part of the same syndrome.

It is important too, that passage of food through the digestive tract be prompt. What speeds up intestinal transit? Eating plenty of vegetable fibre! Not only do the indigestible remains provide greater volume, *more importantly*; the friendly bacteria get a rich nutritive diet too. Friendly bacteria are *methanogens*. They are the ones that produce methane in the gut. They thrive, multiply fast, and greatly increase the bulk of the faeces.

Get this right and:

* bowel movements will occur one to two times a day

* the transit time is greatly reduced

Eating naturally ensures that the sewer pipes are kept well flushed out!

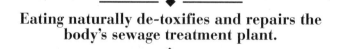

**Eating naturally de-toxifies and repairs the
body's sewage treatment plant.**

How We Eat
Proper Food Combining
The Need for Separating What We Eat

Our digestive system can be thought of as a chemical processing plant. It has to break down into their useful component parts a variety of different 'feedstocks' each requiring a different process. The processes are often conflicting:

- an alkali environment/an acid environment

- a dose of enzyme A/a dose of enzyme B

- pre-treatment in the stomach/immediate treatment in the small intestine

Remarkably, our digestive system can perform these feats, *but not simultaneously*. A chemical engineer would say that each feedstock has to be treated on its own *as a batch*.

For example, a mixed hamper of washing might comprise greasy overalls and silk underwear.

One knows to treat this load in batches because the processes required are conflicting.

We know that the washing machine can satisfy all these requirements on condition that each type of wash is dealt with separately.

The foregoing consideration leads to the concept of *eating food in batches*, which require the same chemical and mechanical treatment in the digestive tract. It is known as the principle of *proper food combining*.

Today we have complicated and confounded the process by introducing new types of food into our diet. Notably starches, dairy products and fruits with a drastically distorted sugar profile.

Foodstuffs can be classified, as can laundry, into the categories which have to be considered independently.

The latest understanding of the biological processes gives the following important results.

- **Fruits** should not be eaten in combination with any of the other categories, particularly protein. Fruits should be eaten on an empty stomach.

1st Reason: fruits are digested in the small intestine, and shouldn't get held up waiting in the stomach. If this happens, they will start to ferment, interfere with other digestive processes, and have their nutritive value compromised.

2nd Reason: fruits have a predominantly acid nature. Acid inhibits ptyalin production in the mouth, thus conflicting with starch requirements and inhibits gastric acid production in the stomach, thus conflicting with protein requirement.

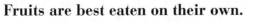

Fruits are best eaten on their own.

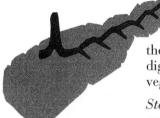

• **Protein/Starch** combinations should be avoided.

1st Reason: the human digestive system is designed for the through-put of a high volume of low density, easily digestible foodstuff, chiefly plant food, i.e., fruit, salads and vegetables.

Starches present a problem since their digestion starts in the mouth (with ptyalin). This digestion is stopped by the acid in the stomach, and then continued in the small intestine, under the action of enzymes like *amylase* secreted down the pancreatic duct by the pancreas.

Pancreas

Proteins, and particularly animal proteins, present another problem They undergo a prolonged churning and exposure to the acids and enzymes present in the stomach. It can be several hours before the stomach releases the resulting chyme into the small intestine. The digestion then continues in the small intestine under the action of enzymes like protease, again secreted down the pancreatic duct by the pancreas.

Unlike the chicken, which has three pancreatic ducts, the single human pancreatic duct is a bottleneck. A choice has to be made by the pancreas as to which enzyme to secrete first. If the starch/protein combination contained predominantly starch (90%), or predominantly protein (90%), then the choice is easy, and digestion can proceed as nature intended. If, perversely, the meal is an equal mix of starch and protein, then enzyme secretion by the pancreas is perturbed. The imperfectly digested remains travel with difficulty through the digestive tract. The highly sophisticated machinery of enzyme activity, hormonal feedback and nutrient absorption is perturbed. The balance of the intestinal flora is disturbed. Bad bacteria multiply. Helpful bacteria are discouraged. The intestinal wall can become porous and, as described earlier, bacteria, funguses (such as candida) and undigested food particles travel through the bloodstream, creating mischief wherever they go. Dyspepsia, ulcerated colitis, liver disorders, demineralization, depression of the immune system, candidiasis, allergies, and general bad health can be the result.

The digestive system is designed to work chiefly on fruit and vegetation. Meat is more problematic. Starch is even more so. It simply is not a good idea to give it more than one problematic foodstuff at a time to digest. Here the problem is compounded by the two nutrients having conflicting treatment processes.

———— ◆ ————

Starch/Protein combinations perturb digestive processes.

———— ◆ ————

2nd Reason: proteins, like starch, also provoke the secretion of insulin. When starches are ingested at the same time, insulin secretion is multiplied. All the bad effects of hyperinsulinemia are therefore multiplied.

———— ◆ ————

Starch/Protein combinations increase hyperinsulinemia.

———— ◆ ————

Worse, almost always fat is present in large proportions with protein. This fat gets stored immediately and preferentially into the fat cells.

———— ◆ ————

Starch/Protein combinations multiply the *fattening* effect of fat.

———— ◆ ————

Finally, let's keep things in perspective. There are many times when *small* amounts of protein are included in a starch dish. Such is the case with traditional Asian cooking where there are little bits of chicken, nuts or fish in the rice. Conversely there are occasions when there are small amounts of starch in a protein dish, like a few bits of sweetcorn in a tuna salad. This is unimportant provided either the starch or the protein dominates. The trouble arises when the proteins and starches are equally balanced and they fight each other for priority. This is the case with so much of what we eat today. For example, bacon and eggs with French fries, hot dogs, hamburgers or cheese sandwich.

———— ◆ ————

Starch/Protein combinations cause trouble when they are present in nearly equal proportions.

———— ◆ ————

* **Salads and Vegetables** do not require any special combining measures.

* **Oils and Fats** do not require any special combining measures.

Timing: Allow these minimum periods after the meal, if you are changing to another category with the next meal:

After **Fruit**, 15 minutes; after **Starch**, 1 hour; after Soft[8] **Protein**, 2 hours; after Hard[8] **Protein**, 3 hours.

The Bottom Line For Food Combining		
Favorable Combinations		
Fruits	mix well with	Fruits
Fruits	mix tolerably well with	Vegetables
Vegetables	mix well with	Proteins
Vegetables	mix well with	Starches
Poor Combinations		
Starches	mix badly with	Fruit
Starches	mix badly with	Protein
Proteins	mix badly with	Starches
Proteins	mix badly with	Fruits

8 Soft proteins are largely of vegetable origin. Hard Proteins are largely of animal origin. See Tables 1 to 5 in Chapter Ten, *Ten Steps to Success*

The Importance of Small and Frequent Meals ('Browsing')

The human anatomy is designed to work with frequent but small quantities of food. The functioning of the stomach, as it receives food and processes it, has been closely studied. One thing is clear. The stomach does not operate as a kind of simmering witches cauldron, where all that is ingested at a meal is all churned up together.

What actually happens is that the first mouthfuls slide down the stomach wall and settle at the far end, the antrum. They fill up the space shown in area 1 of the diagram. Here, muscular churning takes place to thoroughly mix the food with the gastric juices.

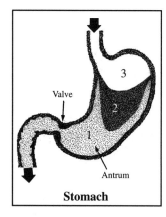

Stomach

The next batch also slides down the stomach wall, partly stays clinging to it, and settles on top of the first batch. This batch too gets good exposure to the gastric juices secreted by the stomach wall. As the first batch is evacuated toward the duodenum, the second is propelled by peristaltic action to take its place in the antrum and to be churned in its turn.

If you stop eating at this point, then digestion has proceeded as it is designed to do. However, for most of us that is not the end of the matter. We are by now only on to the main course. Maybe it is steak and french fries. These slide down into the stomach. Remember that the first and second batches have coated the stomach walls. This third batch settles in the middle (area 2 of the diagram). It is not in contact with the gastric juices. This is the opportunity for the animal meat to putrefy and the potato to ferment.

Many people than add insult to injury by eating fresh fruit desert. This sits on top of everything else you have eaten (area 3 in the diagram). The fruit quietly ferments provoking yet more gas and indigestion.

Here are major reasons why large meals are at the origin of bad digestion and bad health.

——— ◆ ———

Large meals compromise good digestion and undermine health.

——— ◆ ———

It is estimated that the ideal volume of a meal is no more than one and a half pints. This is the volume which just fills the stomach without stretching it. Increase the quantity to two pints and the stomach has to stretch but within acceptable limits. Most of us in the opulent West have been so used to overfilling our stomachs that they have become permanently stretched and out of shape.

The lesson is that we should eat little but often - and always within the principles of Natural Eating!

——— ◆ ———

Eat Naturally - little but often

——— ◆ ———

Chapter Six

The Method

"Human history becomes more and more a race between education and catastrophe." – H. G. Wells

Now that you are Convinced

This chapter sets out the 'Golden Rules' of Natural Eating. They present, in summary form, the chief principles. These rules represent an ideal. It is possible to work towards this ideal in stages. Chapter Ten, *The Ten Steps to Success*, shows how.

After all, we only have so much will-power and motivation, and it is best to focus on the activities that yield the most benefit.

Note that if you already have some diet-susceptible disease such as diabetes or diverticulosis, then some of the priorities could change. Look ahead in Chapter Eight, *The Food/Disease Connection*, and see which of the recommendations you need to work on first.

Restructuring a Way of Thinking

How does this new way of eating work in practice? The first thing to accept is that it *is a new way of eating!* A firm resolve has to be made to swim against the tides of cultural tradition, commercial vested interests, family indoctrination and personal habit.

The behavior of ideas has been likened to that of viruses. Ideas float around in the environment waiting for a susceptible brain to colonize. We all carry a baggage of ideas, opinions, beliefs and prejudices that have taken up residence in our minds in a usually haphazard way. New ideas have to fight the current incumbents for a place to be heard. If they are successful they take up residence and modify your behavior. If the ideas are really successful they are fruitful and multiply by getting you to tell other people about it. That is how ideas, sometimes fancifully called 'mind viruses', spread.

Looked in that way, Natural Eating is a concept, *an idea*, that has to vie for your attention with all the opinions, beliefs and prejudices about nutrition that are already entrenched in your mind.

———— ◆ ————

Wipe the slate clean on what you think you know about nutrition. Have the courage to believe it could be wrong!

———— ◆ ————

You have almost certainly been indoctrinated from an early age by the food producers. For generations they have provided attractive educational materials to schools free of charge. The Beef Lobby has convinced you that you stand in mortal danger of protein deficiency. The Milk Lobby asks you "Got Milk?" and makes you feel bad if you aren't giving it to your kids. The Egg Lobby wants you "to go to work on an egg" and so on.

So our instincts to eat these products can be trusted? **Wrong!**

The people, who process food into food products, are engaged in a battle for growth and market share. They are seeking ever more new ways of *processing* food so that it is ever more tasty, more attractive, more complicated - and therefore has a higher added value. This has reached such an extreme that it is almost impossible to find such a prosaic staple as bread which has not been "improved!" That is, denatured, processed and contaminated with all kinds of unwanted extras. If you can find mass produced, commercial bread which is made *only* from coarse ground, whole-wheat flour, yeast and a pinch of salt, like that eaten by scores of generations of our forebears, then tell the world about it.

The same goes for cereals. There is a bewildering range of ever more exotic breakfast cereal invented for our delectation. The harsh reality is that the original goodness found in the bran and wheat germ has been thrown away. These products have been converted from a moderately nutritious foodstuff into an empty calorie sugar-rush.

To make matters worse, years of propaganda by the food processors have conditioned us to think that we haven't eaten breakfast unless one of these cereals has been consumed. It was not so long ago that corn was grown mainly to fatten cattle for market. It was only later that corn was treated to make it consumable by humans and repackaged as breakfast cereal. It is a dubious, but dramatic marketing success story of the last 40 years. Breakfast cereals have moved from being an insignificant niche market in the 1950s to being all-pervasive today. Corn has been successfully repackaged to fatten people as well as cattle.

But now sales are flagging in the West, so they are now using the power of the media to persuade the cornflake-free Latin Americans to change their breakfast habits.

So our instincts to eat these products can be trusted? **No!**

In most families, as you are being brought up, there is an unsubtle indoctrination going on. "You must eat a hearty breakfast!"; "Make sure you get your protein!"; "I don't want our neighbors thinking we can't afford meat!"; "I'm not eating rabbit food!"; "You must have a second portion of this apple pie I've baked for you!"

Examine closely every one of the prejudices with which your parents have molded your ideas about eating. Jettison them if they don't coincide with *the new way of eating!*

We are all hopelessly entrained in the gearwheels of cultural tradition. Any significant meal has to conform to the format of a starter, meat dish main course (with rolls and butter), dessert (sweet), cheese (and biscuits).

Throw overboard the tyranny of this format! It is a recipe for bad combination, overeating and bad insulin reaction.

Get used to the idea that meals can be eaten more frequently. Get used to the idea that meals have to be *unconventional* –and stick to your guns!

Finally, reject the preconceived idea that the best compliment that one can make about a meal is that it is attractive and *tasty*. Resolve instead to think that the best compliment one can make about a meal is that it is *healthy*. There is nothing to stop it being tasty and attractive too, but these are secondary considerations.

Your taste buds, long anesthetized by the highly flavored products of the food industrialists, will wake up and tingle to the joy of long forgotten delicate taste sensations. Be indignant at the cynical presumption that your only interest is in *taste* and not quality or health.

> **Learn to rejoice in the fact that a meal is not**
>
> - *unbalancing your hormones*
> - *reducing your quality of life*
> - *shortening your lifespan*

What to expect

When you start to eat naturally, you are almost certainly making major changes in the structure of how and what you eat. These changes have their repercussions and during the transition phase may be uncomfortable. That is why it can be wise to introduce the changes gradually.

The digestive system will be in a state of shock! For years it has been abused and mistreated. Many of its functions will have shut down. Your new way of eating will bring immediate benefits; proper food combining will start to reduce digestive problems. On the other hand, the increase in roughage from fruit and vegetables will force lazy and atrophied intestinal muscles to limber up and become operational again. Be prepared for bouts of diarrhea or constipation for several weeks. This is normal during the transition period.

During the transition period you will start to lose *excess fat*. That is the good news. The bad news is that as this fat is released into the bloodstream, it will be accompanied by concentrations of pesticides and other pollutants that have built up in the fat tissues. Your body will have to eliminate these unpleasant chemicals. In the meantime, you may well suffer discomfort from their presence in the blood-stream. Be prepared for symptoms such as increased allergy activity during the transition period.

As you will have learned in this book, food is a potent factor for modifying the hormonal balances in the body. As you shift the emphasis on what you eat, particularly from *bad* carbohydrates, you will be modifying your hormonal balances. During the transitional period you may feel the effects of this with mood swings, sweet cravings, headaches, for example. This is normal.

Bowel Movements

Once you are up and running with your restructured way of eating, you will find that bowel movements:

• will occur once to twice a day

• are soft and easy to expel

• do not have a noxious odor

• are copious in quantity

• food will have a rapid transit time through the digestive tract.

These are the normal characteristics of bowel movements in the human species.

When you get to this point you will know for sure that you are eating correctly. You will rejoice at the wholesome feeling of health and tone in your intestines. You will know that the friendly flora and fauna are flourishing. (They are providing most of the bulk in the faeces.)

Know also that instead of having a clogged up sewer system for a gut, it is an efficient toxic waste disposal unit. Instead of hanging around in the intestine creating mischief and undermining general health, the noxious toxic products of digestion are swiftly and efficiently shown the back door.

Flatulence

It is perfectly normal for some air to be swallowed as you eat and for some gases to be formed by bacterial fermentation in the intestines. Under normal Natural Eating circumstances, this gas does not cause discomfort, and is evacuated when you 'pass wind'.

Believe it or not, this process has been measured. On average, wind is passed 13 times a day and has a total volume of about two pints. It does not have a noxious odor.

On the other hand, those Westerners who have really bad eating habits, can pass up to 40 pints per day of noxious smelling gas!

If for example, you have problems with gas, large volumes, wrenching gut pains or noxious smells, then there is something wrong. In view of the appalling eating habits that are commonplace in the West, this is a common problem.

The only *healthy* cure for digestive problems of this kind is to eat in harmony with the way your digestive system is designed to work - i.e. *Naturally!*

Mouth Hygiene

When you eat naturally mouth hygiene is vastly improved.

* due to the stimulation and hardening *(keratisation)* of the gums from the mechanical action of chewing a high volume of raw vegetable matter and,

* From an improvement of saliva quality.

Most people on a Western diet have a completely deregulated saliva composition. The saliva should contain a well-balanced cocktail of enzymes and anti-bacterial agents. Once onto a *Natural* diet, the saliva finds its equilibrium and can fulfill a major role, keeping the mouth sterile, wholesome, and sweet-smelling.

If you have poor dentition, do the best you can to get it fixed. It is surprising how often people are pushed into poor food choices, just because they cannot chew the right foods comfortably.

——————— ◆ ———————

Get your teeth fixed for optimum chewing efficiency.

——————— ◆ ———————

The Consumption Priorities

What are our consumption priorities? The same as those of our Pleistocene ancestors! With the proviso that the devil is in the detail, here are the broad outlines. Lots of fruit and soft vegetation (salads and vegetables); moderate amounts of other 'good' carbohydrates; moderate amounts of vegetable protein; moderate amounts of qualifying animal matter (optional); occasional borderline carbohydrates .

The broad principles are simply said. Our Pleistocene ancestors had incredible jungle survival skills. We have to develop the same level of skill for survival in the supermarket jungle. Let's not forget that there is not a single food that we eat today that would be recognized by our hunter/gatherer forebears of the African savannah. So even when we talk in broad terms about eating fruits, *his* fruits were different species with somewhat different nutrient profiles to our apples, oranges and pears today. That is why we have to be savvy about *everything* we eat and why in this book we go into some detail to explain how even with fruits for example, we have to make wise choices between them.

———— ◆ ————

**The broad principles of Natural Eating are simply said.
The devil is in the detail.**

———— ◆ ————

The following consumption profiles set out the broad priorities.

A. Unrestricted Consumption

There is a totally laudable campaign by most governments in the West to encourage the consumption of "five a day" portions of fruit and vegetables. It shows how lamentably low is current consumption that five a day is considered an improved target. In reality, the target should be closer to *30 portions* per day! Here are the ideal targets for Natural Eating.

Vegetation (Salads, Green and Yellow Vegetables)

Their consumption should be *increased* to a minimum of 40% of the diet. The human species is designed to get a good percentage of protein from vegetation. You have to eat lots, up to 3 pounds net per day (measure it out to start with).That is the way that our bodies are designed.

Fruit

Their consumption should be *increased* to a minimum of 25% of the diet. Again, eat lots. Up to 2 pounds per day. Concentrate on the unrestricted fruits in Table 1 of Appendix 1, *Good Foods to be Eaten in Bulk*.

B. Restricted and Controlled Consumption

Dairy Products

Their consumption should be reduced to very little or zero.

Red Farm Meat

Its consumption should be reduced to as close to zero as possible.

Farm Fowl

Skinless chicken and turkey breast are OK in modest quantities. Consumption of other parts should be reduced as much as possible.

Wild Game

Truly wild game that feeds off what it finds in its natural habitat is OK to consume modestly. It will be low fat and should have a good fatty acid profile. This includes grouse, pigeon, partridge, wild boar, pheasant, venison, rabbit or hare.

Oily Fish

It is good to consume modestly.

Other Seafood

It is OK to consume modestly.

Vegetable Protein (nuts, legumes and meat substitutes)

It is important to consume modest quantities of raw nuts regularly. If you are a vegetarian it is important to eat legumes and meat substitutes modestly. (Because of their anti-nutrients, legumes and soy particularly are not miracle foods.)

Cereals, Sugars and Starches (*bad* and *borderline* carbohydrates. See Tables 4 and 5, Appendix 1)

Their consumption should be restricted as much as possible.

Eggs

It is OK to consume moderately.

Fats and Oils

In today's supermarket it is quite difficult to find plant foods that naturally contain Omega 3 oils. For this reason it is good to use about 1 tbs. per day of canola, walnut, or flax oil as part of a salad dressing for example.

If you are not watching your weight, one additional tablespoon of the Omega 3 oils or olive oil per day may be used.

All other fats and oils – none is best.

Sodium/Potassium Ratio

Avoid all processed foods containing salt. Limit added salt at the table or in cooking. These measures, together with the high consumption of plant food, will ensure that an optimum sodium/potassium ratio is maintained.

Acid/Alkali Ratio

Following the foregoing guidelines will ensure that an optimum acid/alkali ratio will be maintained.

Bottom Line for Consumption Priorities

Eating in this fashion will ensure that the basic parameters of the Natural Eating Pattern (Chapter Three) are observed.

➡ High Volume
➡ High Fibre
➡ Low Calorie Density
➡ High Micronutrient Density
➡ Low Glycemic
➡ Low Fat
➡ Low Salt

These are the broad outlines. It is not necessary to go 'cold turkey' straight away. Chapter Ten, *Ten Steps to Success* shows how to get there in stages. Remember that any movement in the right direction will bring its benefits.

> All movement in the right direction is beneficial.

Hints and tips

Fruit

Tomatoes can be eaten either as a fruit or a salad vegetable. Tomatoes are acid to the digestion. Be aware that starch/tomato combinations (e.g. spaghetti Napoletane or tomato sandwich) could give a digestive difficulty.

Strawberries and raspberries seem to be an exception to the general rule about not combining fruits with other foods. Most people find that strawberries and raspberries do not give a digestive difficulty at the end of a properly combined meal.

Liquidizing fruits into juices is not recommended. Ready made fruit juices are even less recommended. Juicing, pasteurizing, concentrating, reconstituting are processes which

- destroy the nature and utility of the natural fibers and increase the glycemic index.

- destroy many of the essential complex molecules necessary as feedstock for the human chemical factory.

There is a more important point: when we eat an apple, for example, it requires *mastication* and it *takes time*. As a result our brains register the process at its true value, gastric juices are mobilized, and we feel satiated more easily.

Melons and tropical fruits like bananas, papayas, mangoes, although fruits, are high in sucrose and starch. Due to their high glycemic index, they should be consumed only modestly.

Some people find it helps to avoid mixing sweet fruits (bananas, fresh dates) with other fruits, particularly acid fruits (citrus, tomato, berries).

Melons are best eaten alone, not with other fruit. But keep matters in proportion. If you find a piece of melon in a fruit salad, it's probably not a big deal. Melons (all kinds) are *bad* carbohydrates, but low density ones. You should not be eating lots at a sitting anyway.

Many people have digestive difficulties if they drink on top of fruit. Definitely avoid drinking tea as it contains 'anti-nutrients' that reduce the bio-availability of nutrients to the body.

The Golden Rules For Natural Eating
(In Ideal Terms)

1. The food to which as a species we are primarily adapted is soft vegetation and fruit. Think *Big* when planning volumes of fruit and vegetables. Up to 2 pounds of fruit per day. Up to 3 pounds of salads and colored vegetables per day. Put vegetables at the center of the plate.

2. Keep meals *simple*. The fewer items the better.

3. Eat a minimum of one large salad per day and one pound of fruit per day.

4. Prefer raw vegetables to cooked. When cooking prefer steaming, baking or stir-frying.

5. Calories, no need to count them. You can eat to satiety provided these rules are followed. Your body, now receiving the correct fuel supply, can do the rest.

6. Restrict all *bad* carbohydrates. Be wary of anything that comes in a packet, tin, jar, bottle or box. Read the Fine Print! Consult the Glycemic Index Tables, Appendix 1.

7. Restrict red or fatty meat and their products. (Table 1, Chapter 10.) Limit the consumption of other hard but acceptable proteins (Table 2, Chapter 10.) Concentrate on sources of 'good' proteins (Tables 3 – 5, Chapter 10.) Don't overeat protein.

8. Limit the consumption of dairy products. Ban them if there are signs of intolerance.

9. Be frugal with fats and oils. Replace *bad* fats and oils (See Chapter Five) with Canola oil. Walnut and flax oils are also fine. Be cautious with cheese.

10. Favor *good* desserts. Return to the thinking that cakes, pastries, puddings, tarts, ice-cream etc. are luxuries to be consumed on red-letter days, like in olden times!

11. A well combined meal is either

    - uniquely fruit

    - uniquely salads and vegetable

    - vegetable with a small side-order of *good starch*

    - vegetable with a small side order of *good protein*

12. Avoid processed foods containing salt. Avoid the use of salt in cooking. Limit the use of salt at the table.

When changing from one category of food to another, allow these times to elapse.	
After **Fruit**	15 mn
After **Starch**	1 hr
After *Soft* **Protein**	2 hrs
After *Hard* **Protein**	3 hrs

Cooked fruit generally becomes a *bad* carbohydrate and combines and digests like one. Even so, many people have difficulty digesting even cooked fruit in combination with starch or protein. Be aware that the starch/fruit combination of apple pie, for example, could be at the origin of a digestive difficulty.

Dried fruit (raisins, sultanas, currants and dried dates, figs, apricots, peaches etc.) are to be treated as sugar/starches both from a food combining viewpoint and from a *bad* carbohydrate viewpoint. Nevertheless, eaten in modest quantities they are a good source of concentrated nourishment. The drying process has, of course, destroyed many of the complex essential molecules, so in no way can dried fruit be a substitute for the fresh variety.

Vegetable Proteins

Treat nuts and legumes (lentils, peanuts, beans, soy bean) as *proteins*. They are further classified as *soft* proteins. Legumes are a useful addition to the Natural Eater's nutrition. Eat legumes in small portions and dilute them by eating with a large volume of vegetables.

Drinking

Don't worry too much about drinking lots of water. On this régime you'll be getting four pints just from the fruit and vegetables.

It *is* possible to drink both water and dry wine with a meal. The stomach simply pours in more acid to compensate for the dilution. If you notice digestive difficulties, however, don't do it any more! Don't even think of drinking fruit juices, sugary colas/sodas or beer with a meal.

Processed Food

Eat food that is the least processed as possible. Processing destroys fibers and leaches out micro-nutrients such as phytochemicals, minerals and vitamins. Processing increases the glycemic index. Processing almost always means the addition of seemingly endless lists of unwanted, useless and often harmful compounds such as coloring, artificial flavorings, preservatives, emulsifiers, stabilizers, fungicides, pesticides, sugars, salt, sulfur, hydrogenated fat and a variety of junk fillers like whey, modified starch and unbleached wheat flour. Even *water* is injected to plump up the volume of products like ham, bacon and chicken breasts!

Potato

So far in the book, this tuber has been comprehensively disparaged. This is deliberate. The potato, like a cuckoo in the nest, has pushed overboard the rightful occupants of our diet – green plant foods. It has only taken a couple of hundred years to do so but the consequences for the population's health are dramatic. Incredibly, average Americans now get their vitamin C mostly from French fries. At what cost? High intakes of *bad* fats, empty calories and blood sugar out of control.

That is the dark side of the picture. Is there no place then for the potato? It does have one saving grace. When it is boiled or steamed it has a low carbohydrate density. It is still a *bad* carbohydrate, and it is still strongly insulinemic[1] but the healthy person has to eat a fair portion to trip the glycemia threshold. This opens up possibilities. A potato in a soup to thicken it will be acceptable. When you are confident that you have got consumption of potato under control, enjoy the occasional meal that is accompanied by a few boiled new potatoes. Take care not to eat any other *bad* carbohydrates at the same meal.

Know What You Are Eating

Take your fine reading glasses with you to the supermarket. Even health food stores are not safe. *Read the food labels.* Ruthlessly extirpate the bad carbohydrates. Shy away from products that have lengthy ingredient lists. Avoid oils and fat additives, particularly animal fats and hydrogenated fats.

———————— ◆ ————————

Know What You Are Eating. Read The Fine print!

———————— ◆ ————————

Caffeine

Caffeine provokes the secretion of insulin. Prefer decaffeinated drinks wherever possible. See Chapter Seven, *Top Ten Topics.*

Candies

Dark, bitter, chocolate, preferably with a minimum of 70% cocoa, is safe to eat modestly at the end of a meal. The little, individually wrapped square of dark bitter chocolate served at the end of a meal in classy restaurants is fine.

Who is Natural Eating For?

The short answer is everybody! However I don't expect you to be satisfied with such a laconic response, so let us look at the longer answers for various interest groups. Everybody should read the next section on babies/toddlers. Not only does it set the tone for everything that follows, it will guide you in your relations with those who do, even if you do not have a baby of your own.

Baby/toddler

Up to the age of about three years old, human babies are lactivores (see Chapter Four). They are designed to work on human breast milk. In primitive societies, babies are not weaned until they are about three years old, although solid foods, partially pre-masticated by their mothers, are

---

1 That is, the potato generates a production of insulin out of proportion to that predicted by its glycemic index.

introduced slowly from about 12 months.

That is the ideal. But what to do in the modern world? Mercifully, the movement towards breast-feeding has made this practice not only acceptable but also practicable. Today, mothers can give breast to their child in public places, something unthinkable 50 years ago.

Of course it is unthinkable in the West for the vast majority of mothers to breast feed after about 12 months, let alone to pre-masticate pap for a two year old. So what is there to be done?

Fortunately, the companies that make formula milk are getting cuter about making a product that imitates human milk as closely as possible. They have come a long way in 50 years. No more cow milk allergens; a much better ratio of fats to proteins and a much better composition of vitamins, minerals and essential fatty acids.

They do not, however, mimic the fact that the composition of mother's milk changes as the baby gets older. For example, in the first weeks of life, a baby cannot utilize the essential fatty acids, linoleic acid and alpha-linolenic acid. During this time, the mother's milk contains compounds that compensate for this.

Secondly, the mother's milk contains antibodies and other compounds that protect the baby from disease early in life. Again, formula milk cannot provide these.

So the message is, breast feed if you can, and for as long as you can. Then move onto, and supplement with, the best formula milk you can find.

What about solid foods? The first principle has to be, eat naturally! The more the baby eats in accordance with the general principles enunciated in this book, the better.

The second principle is, people like to eat what they have always eaten. The best start in life that you can give your baby is to give him the *taste* for healthy foods. Get him used to eating healthy foods at this stage, and that *liking* will stay with him for life.

––––––– ◆ –––––––

Get your baby used to healthy foods, and that liking will stay with him for life.

––––––– ◆ –––––––

The first good habit to instill is, yes, the eating of vegetables. No need to make special arrangements, just take what you, as a Natural Eater, eat every day and reduce down to a form appropriate to the child's stage of development. Today's food processors are a good substitute for the masticating jaws of the mother, but no one knows yet if the absence of the mother's saliva is significant.

Essential lifelong habit number one: eat vegetation every day.

The next solid to be introduced is fruit. Why not *fruit* first of all? It is a question of strategy. Better to get your child used to the bland taste of vegetables before introducing the sweeter and jazzier taste of grapes, bananas, tangerines, apples, pears, cherries, peaches etc. In the early stages, make sure that fruits are skinned and pipped. Give fruits to your baby every day. This is the second essential eating habit to instill for life. Eat fruit every day.

Essential lifelong habit number two: eat fruit every day.

What about meat? The same remark applies as for adults. The problem for meat eaters today is that there is nothing available resembling the animal matter for which we are genetically programmed. Of course many people bring their children up perfectly successfully as vegetarians. But if you do not want to go that far, then fish and the occasional fowl are OK. Just remember, you don't have to give your child anything that, as a Natural Eater, you would not eat yourself.

There will certainly be times when it is just not possible to prepare your own baby food. What about the commercially available products? Here again the food manufacturers have got a lot cleverer about formulating reasonably healthy substitutes. When you go shopping the same rules apply. Take your reading glasses and scrutinize the Ingredient Lists.

Don't be misled by the large, attractive marketing labels proclaiming "healthy," "low-fat," "no artificial additives" etc. The food manufacturers always put the advantages of their product in large attractive lettering. The truth is grudgingly portrayed in the smallest legally allowable print in an obscure corner of the label.

This time you are reading the ingredient list for a vulnerable, dependent, baby, so be conscientious! Don't buy anything which contains ingredients that you would not want for yourself. Watch out for all the baddies: salt, sugar, glucose syrup, vegetable oil, fat, starch etc.

There will be other times when you are drawn into feeding your child starches like bread and pasta. A little of each every day is not a problem, but always insist on the whole-wheat version. Whole-wheat spaghetti is particularly acceptable. The other types of pasta are borderline glycemic, but are still not as bad as bread.

Boiled potatoes are OK too in modest quantities. The big no-nos are French fries and potato chips. As ever, keep the emphasis on a high consumption of fruit and vegetation relative to the starches.

Finally, drinks. You know the answer already! If he is not drinking his mother's milk or formula milk, then the only other he should have is *plain water.* Just about all the alternatives are *plain bad*. All? What about fruit juice? Well, if you have squeezed it yourself, this is tolerable in modest quantities. But it is not good for a baby to be quaffing volumes of fruit juice. It gives a sugar rush and helps rot teeth. Carrot juice too is highly glycemic; avoid it. Other vegetable juices, or better still, vegetable soup can be fine. But why bother? Get your child to accept water as the normal thirst quencher, and you have saved yourself trouble and given him a good lifestyle reflex.

Essential lifelong habit number three: quench thirst with water.

Will any kind of water do? Tap-water, unjustly, is much maligned and is quite safe to use when boiled. For all young babies, the water should be boiled anyway. For the cautious, by all means buy bottled water. Avoid the high sodium brands; distilled is the safest.

As for packaged drinks be ultra-suspicious. Read the fine print. They are almost always loaded with sugar and other nasties. Don't even think of giving your child colas and other carbonated drinks.

Don't forget, this is one phase in your child's life when he is most open to influence from adults. It is now that you have to indoctrinate him with good consumption reflexes. You routinely take your baby to be inoculated against diseases. This is the time to inoculate him too with some benign, life preserving 'mind-viruses'.

This is *not* the time to introduce him to pizzas, hamburgers, take-away chicken or hot-dogs. Even less is it the time to introduce your child to candies, cookies, ice cream and confectionery! If you can get him through this phase without ever having tasted them, then you are well on the way to insulating him from addiction later on. Better for him and the whole family not to have them in the house at all.

Essential Lifelong habit number four: make your home a junk food-free zone

At a later stage, he will learn to exercise self-discipline and, like a socially responsible drinker, be able to consume just enough for the pleasure without compromising health. Your baby is not old enough to know about postponing self-gratification, so you have to provide the discipline for him.

The hard part is with friends and relatives. They want to give 'treats'. Worse, ingratiate themselves with the child. They don't understand, and don't even cooperate with your stance. When they ask ," Mind if I give him a candy?", you respond, with a perfectly straight face,"I would rather you gave him a tot of gin!"

It is being realized that many adult health problems are laid down in these formative years. Perhaps the most significant is *obesity*. If your baby is allowed to get overweight, then the chances are that he will be overweight or even obese, for the rest of his life. Worse, if your baby is overweight, he is already laying down plaque in his arteries, storing up a mid-life heart attack.

How do you avoid your baby getting fat? Just the same way as adults avoid it. It is a theme that runs right though this book. Eating naturally eliminates the risk of getting overweight. For a summary of the guidelines refer to the segment "Overweight/Obesity" in Chapter Eight.

Children/Adolescents

The special needs of children and adolescents are often exaggerated. They will be eating a lot for their size, but they do not need any particular divergence from the Natural Eating Pattern. By far the greatest problem is to stop them from eating harmful foods!

It is too much to expect that you can, like the little Dutch boy with his finger in the dike, hold back the floodwaters of the junk food society. Accept with good grace that your child will eat junk food from time to time, but don't be defeatist! Make sure that at home he is eating naturally. The most important thing you can do is ensure that he has the ballast to keep his ship of nutritional health steady. If that is solidly assured, then he will survive the storms of junk food relatively unscathed.

Avoid using junk food as a treat, much less as a reward. You are surely making a rod for your own back if you use candies as incentives.

――――― ◆ ―――――

Never use junk foods as a reward or incentive.

――――― ◆ ―――――

Rather, you need to indoctrinate children with the idea that junk food is shoddy, tacky, malignant, even hazardous, toxic and poisonous. Children will accept that they are different from their peers if it is presented as their particular belief-system. They need to be given the arguments and words to use when their eating habits come under question. Let them read this book. Let them understand that they are eating in a way that not only provides all the nutrients they need, they are avoiding the deficiency diseases of their peers.

Play hardball. If necessary, discreetly draw attention to the signs in their peers of deficiency disease, malnutrition and over-indulgence: the poor complexion, the acne and pimples, the constant colds and flu, the dull, listless eyes, the allergies and eczema, the bad breath and body odor, the lack of physical fitness and the grossness of obesity. You may have scruples against this approach, but you have to think that your child is being peddled temptations that are even more pervasive than those offered by the neighborhood drug dealer.

Does this mean that your child should never have a hamburger, cola, ice-cream or candy? Of course not! If you have done your job well, the child will be sensible and will be able to handle social situations adroitly. He will still want to go to birthday parties and proms, and to hang out at the local burger joint. He will want to be part of the scene. But this is where he will need the self-discipline, confidence and social skills to limit the potential damage.

At home, you have an iron responsibility to ensure that the right foodstuffs are constantly available. Always have a supply of ready-to-eat fruit, vegetables and salads. Have homemade dishes like vegetable hot-pot, lentil soup and ratatouille, available in the fridge and freezer. Have stocks of frozen veggie burgers, soy protein hot dogs and oily fish. Lay in stocks of canned salmon, sardines and tuna, as well as tomatoes and baked beans and of certain vegetables like palm hearts, artichoke hearts and water chestnuts. Never run out of whole-wheat spaghetti and whole-grain rye and barley.

In other words have a larder well-stocked for Natural Eating. Water should still be the main drink. Try carbonated with a twist of lemon. Make up your own lemonade (no sugars!). Later on, tea iced or otherwise, is OK. Finally, remind yourself that a child needs a role model. From the youngest age, if he sees the feeding patterns of the adult Natural Eaters, he will want to emulate them. He will find that lifestyle the most normal.

Get your child into the habit of filling up with food at home, and of preparing and taking food supplies with him when he goes out. Never have junk foods in the house. Never buy cookies, cakes, pastries, candies, hamburgers, hot-dogs, ice-cream, pizzas, or ready made meals. Never have colas, fruit juices, or carbonated drinks in the house.

What about condiments? It's been said that the only way to get a kid to eat his vegetables is to smother them in ketchup. Strangely, if that is what works, then this is OK. A good quality ketchup (read the ingredient list) is not such a bad condiment. The main draw-back is the sugar content. But, for a Natural Eater, ketchup used in *modest* quantities is a small and tolerable lapse. Better still, make up your own ketchup – a recipe is given in the Natural Eating Manual. Likewise for Worcester sauce and various brown sauces (read the ingredient list!).

Don't forget herbs and spices. They are full of healthful phyto-chemicals (hence their pungent taste and aroma). We are fortunate that today we have access to a huge variety of herbs and spice. Often they are available freshly growing or at least freshly cut. Get into the habit of using copious quantities of natural herbs and spices in all your dishes. Wean yourself and your family off processed and junk sauces.

Pregnant and Nursing Women

All we know about how our bodies work, and how our pre-historic ancestors evolved, shows that no special departure from the Natural Eating Pattern is indicated. Really, what about extra calcium? Our ancestors never knew anything about calcium. Certainly we have no instincts to search out calcium-rich foods. But if that doesn't convince you, studies show that calcium supplementation does not make one jot of difference to calcium metabolism.

Read what happens with a pregnant and nursing woman. The mother's body meets the demand for extra calcium by three *hormonal* activities. First, the intestines absorb a *higher percentage* of calcium from the ordinary foods that she eats. Secondly the kidneys become *more efficient* at recycling calcium recovered from the urine. Thirdly some calcium is *borrowed* from the bones. Nothing that the mother eats, supplements, or does changes this process.

As soon as menstruation restarts, the bone density recovers. Nothing the women does in the way of supplementation speeds up or changes this process! The main lesson to draw from this is to space your pregnancies so as to allow full recovery to take place.

Of course your doctor will be prescribing all kinds of dietary supplements. There is not the space in this book to explain, one by one, why these supplements are not necessary so you will dutifully take them. Just know that the pregnant Natural Eater need have no fear of having dietary deficiencies. For example, one of the latest vitamins to be recommended for pregnant women is folic acid. The diet of the average American woman is deficient in it. But where is folic acid found? *In foliage!* The Natural Eater mother will be absorbing high levels of folic acid in her salads and 'SuperVeg[2]', - as well as all the other essential nutrients for her baby.

On the contrary, it is ever more important to not consume all the contraindicated foods like *bad* fats and oils and *bad* carbohydrates.

Finally, what about the cravings and nauseas of morning sickness? This is very definitely a tough time for the pregnant woman. Her hormonal messengers have just been given a new set of orders, and they are running around in confusion. Messages are late arriving or don't arrive at all. Some messengers stray into enemy territory and start an uprising or get liquidated. Worse, there are two generals in charge of the army, the woman's own body and the fetus which is already manipulating the woman's hormones to serve its own purposes.

What should she do? The truth is, not a lot. This is a time for going with the flow. It is a case of any port in a storm. She eats when she can and she eats what she can bear to eat. No point in getting neurotic about bizarre

2 SuperVeg is the term often used to describe a class of particularly healthful vegetables. They include most brassicas. See Table 6 in Chapter Ten, The Ten Steps to Success.

or absent appetites. Just relax and wait for this phase to pass. The fetus will make sure he gets all he needs, robbing if need be, his mother's own stores. This will also be a time to take the vitamin and mineral supplements prescribed by the doctor. This is one occasion when 'double-guessing' nature is a legitimate strategy to bolster the mother's nutrient intake.

Thirty-Something

This is likely to be a phase of life when health will seem good and there is no need to concern yourself about the future. The reality is that it is this period of life when you need to set the scene for your later years. Bad eating habits now quickly lead to obesity, heart disease and diabetes. They lay down the foundation for the degenerative diseases of middle and old age like arthritis, rheumatism and even Alzheimer's.

It is at this age that the blood sugar control mechanism starts to shows its age. It copes less well with the stress that we put on it. It is now that 'middle-age spread' begins to show. This is your warning that you are pre-diabetic. Take it seriously. Take your eating pattern in hand. Relieve your body of that sugar-stress by following the guidelines in this book.

But most importantly of all, this is the last chance to build up bone density capital. Read the chapters on osteoporosis in Chapter Eight, *The Food/Disease Connection*. Remember, it is not a question of eating calcium tablets. Bone health is all about eating in such a way as to marshal your body's hormonal messengers into laying down calcium in the right places – your bones – and not in the wrong places – your arteries, kidneys and joints.

The Menopausal Woman

Menopausal changes start in the early forties, building up to the finality around the age of 50. As with pregnancy, this is a time when a woman's hormones are undergoing a major reshuffle. It is therefore *potentially* a period when Western women will have those familiar symptoms of hot flushes, irritability, hypersensitivity, depression, tension headaches and night sweating. However, in most simple societies, (such as peasant Greek and Mayan) these symptoms are almost unknown. Indeed, many women in the West do not suffer them either. What makes the difference?

Not surprisingly, the main drug influencing hormonal balances is *food*. The bodily dysfunctions caused by dietary errors will be *amplified* during menopause. Controlled studies showed that a diet rich in bio-flavonoids and vitamin C provided complete relief for two-thirds of the women and partial relief for a further 20%. Where are bioflavonoids and vitamin C found? In fruit and vegetation! Just this one simple change, boosting the intake of fruit and vegetation, is enough to dramatically reduce the disagreeable symptoms of menopause. And don't forget that *bad* carbohydrates and *bad* fats (Chapter Five) have a major effect on hormonal balances. Getting these right will help enormously too. Lesson? *Eliminate dietary errors!* In other words, eat naturally.

Is this all? Not quite. There are other, secondary, dimensions such as the stress of the Western way of life, the psychological finality of becoming infertile and the tension in relationships caused by changes (either up or down) in libido. There is a strong mind/body connection. Just know that managing stress and psychological moods will also help stabilize hormonal balances.

So much for negotiating the menopausal climax. What about the long term? What about osteoporosis and heart disease? These are both major problems for post-menopausal women, but only in the West! By the time you have finished reading this book, you will have learned, through several repetitions, that these are optional diseases. Get your eating patterns right, cut out smoking, and get on with life without a worry for these conditions.

Finally, what about hormone replacement therapy (HRT)? We can be fairly confident that Pleistocene grandmothers did not distill pregnant horses' urine to obtain estrogen-rich extracts. There is no reason from a purely health point of view why a menopausal Natural Eater should supplement with estrogen.

On the other hand there are dimensions to HRT, such as its reputation for retarding the outward signs of aging. These are matters that are beyond the scope of this book and a woman who is interested in those aspects should make that decision in consultation with her health professional.

The Elderly

It is at this time of life that eating naturally can bring some of the most rapid relief to distressing ailments like stiff joints, arthritis, digestive upsets and general ill-health. See Chapter Eight. These are the ailments that emerge, like the wreck of a ship, as the tide recedes. For a great part of our lives, our body's biochemistry has sufficient 'redundancy' built into its system to patch around errors of lifestyle. With old age, these margins of error have disappeared. Now more than ever, it is important to harmonize how you eat with the needs of your body. When you do so, then many of those troublesome maladies disappear.

Eating naturally is the ideal, of course. There are no other special measures to take. Just make sure that your dentition, whether original or artificial, is working efficiently. Many old people eat badly simply because they choose foods that don't need chewing. As an older person, do make sure that you are eating the proper rations of fruit, salads and vegetables.

Surveys show that older people, who tend to have less efficient digestive systems anyway, skimp on these foods. As a result they, and their immune systems, are deficient in anti-oxidants and other essential micro-nutrients.

Get that right and you'll live out your years in good shape!

Vegetarians and Vegans

Many people, who take up vegetarianism, make the mistake of simply eliminating animal matter from their *normal*, eat-anything, diet. As a result, some vegetarians and vegans are obese, have poor complexions and suffer ill health simply because they are continuing with the other bad habits. Notably, the consumption of cereals, bread, pasta and other complex carbohydrates. There will be other errors too, like the use of dairy products and the bad fats and oils.

Vegetarians and vegans will find in the pages of this book exactly the right prescription for eating healthily. All that you have to do is to eat naturally, ignoring the animal products where they are mentioned, and think of the vegetable alternatives instead.

Veganism is a very healthy lifestyle, provided that the Natural Eating consumption pattern is carefully followed. The secret is to eat more like the gorilla (a natural vegan) - very high volumes of plant material. See the Table in 'The Stolid Gorilla', Chapter Three.

Some vegans worry about the one micro-element that is never found in plant food -Vitamin B_{12}. There is still a lot of debate about whether the B_{12} made in the intestine by bacteria is bio-available. For a gorilla it is, but for humans this has yet to be proved. Studies on vegans show that their bodies are remarkably good at recycling waste B_{12} for periods up to at least 10 years. The quantities required by the body are absolutely minute – less than one microgram per day. It is thought that many vegans derive sufficient B_{12} just from biological contamination of homegrown vegetables, as is suspected with certain long-established Iranian peasant vegan sects. Whatever the truth of the matter, a vegan should make double sure by supplementing with a 2 mcg tablet of vitamin B_{12} once a week. Vegetarians will get all they need from the occasional egg and cheese.

———— ◆ ————

**The Natural Eating Pattern is the ideal
formula for a vegetarian or vegan régime.**

———— ◆ ————

C h a p t e r   S e v e n

Top Ten Topics

1. Genetically Modified Foods (GMFs)

Most of what we eat is already genetically modified, by hundreds, sometimes thousands, of years of hybridization and cross breeding, and it has rarely been an improvement from a nutritional point of view. For example, farm animal meat is worse than the meat of the wild creatures from which they are descended, and high glycemic carrots would be unrecognizable to a Roman, who only ate the carrot-tops anyway.

Large swathes of our food supply have already been genetically modified in the wrong direction. Now, genetic engineering speeds up the process thousands of times.

---◆---

Genetic engineering magnifies the distortions from our ideal food supply.

---◆---

Genetic engineering also introduces genes from species that have nothing to do with each other like fish genes going into tomatoes. Furthermore, anyone who works with genes knows that they are multipurpose. For example, in humans the gene for fair hair also controls for introverted personality. What could be a more unexpected side effect?

Genetic scientists are playing with an immensely powerful tool, the ramifications of which are only partly understood in the best of times.

The worrying aspect is this. Genetic modification is driven by agro-industry. Their motives are driven by money. They want to create products that have an advantage over their rivals. Their products have to be *patentable* so that they can be sure to get the development costs back and make a decent profit.

No agro-industrialist is interested in organic foods. There is nothing to patent and even less to sell! Genetically modified foods are all to do with convenience of production (like extended shelf life, or herbicide resistance) and nothing to do with nutrient value.

For example, when they genetically modify a potato to be pest resistant, what do they do? They give it genes that cause it to make insecticides!

This is so the farmer can save on pesticides and even claim that he has used a lot less in the cultivation. For all we know, a consumer could be eating more pesticides than if they had been sprayed on.

Governments and the industry hasten to reassure the public that GMFs are safe. But that is not the point! Volcanic ash might be safe to eat, but is it food? Of course not, and that is why GMF should be opposed. Already our current food supply is too far removed from our naturally adapted profile. Genetic modification is taking it even further away.

───────── ◆ ─────────

Genetic Modification is taking us ever further away from our naturally adapted food supply.

───────── ◆ ─────────

The question is a very fundamental one. The Natural Eater should have nothing to do with genetically engineered products. We are organic creatures that have grown up in harmony with a particular pattern of naturally occurring vegetation and fauna. We are certainly not robots designed to run on the artificial creations of the bio-tech lab.

In the meantime, how do you know if you are consuming genetically modified food? The scandal is that mostly you can't find out. The current FDA policy states that there is no need for special labeling.

The European Union (EU) is introducing a system of labeling for genetically engineered products. Meanwhile unmarked American GMFs, like soy bean products, tomato paste and corn (maize) products have been slipping in unremarked into the EU market.

To their credit, the Europeans, and particularly the British, have been scandalized by this infiltration of their food supply by the "Frankenstein creations" of agro-industry. Encouragingly, the outcry has been so great that major supermarkets and fast food chains are hastening to declare themselves GMF-free zones. Their purchasing departments scour the world to locate non-GMF suppliers. The pressure is so great that many large suppliers in the United States are scrambling to retrieve lost markets by paying a premium to farmers for guaranteed non-GMF products.

2. Bread

The decline in the quality of bread since the invention of the steel roller mill in the 1870s, and more particularly since World War II, is one of the saddest episodes in mass nutrition. Bread should be made from fresh, rough-ground whole wheat (or rye) flour, yeast and *nothing else!*

Today the supermarket shelves groan with a vast variety of breads. Almost without exception they are bad for your health. Until things improve, you can safely ignore these shelves. What is wrong with this bread?

The first problem came with the spread of the steel roller mill at the end of the 19th Century. Grains milled with these machines are turned into a much finer flour with the texture of talcum powder. What is the advantage of that? For the manufacturer it leads to a fluffier and more predictable baking bread. Unfortunately, the process also breaks open the starch granules. This gives the bread a much higher glycemic index. Result? Modern bread, although cheaper and fluffier than ever before, is a Trojan horse silently undermining your health. Remember the "hyperinsulinemia iceberg" in Chapter Five? Every time you eat bread today remember the Titanic!

Second, most of the goodness in bread is in the bran and wheat-germ. The trouble for bread manufacturers is that these nutrients make bread unpredictable and variable in quality. So they take them out and throw them away! Nowadays, governments have realized that this impoverishes the food supply of the people, so they ordain that certain minerals and vitamins be added to the white flour.

The problem is that there are thousands of different complex molecules in the discarded material. Not only is the government unable to specify more than a tiny fraction, these compounds need to be present *together* for them to be effective nutritionally. Just with this action alone the bread has been transformed from the staff of life, an important food since biblical times, into an *empty*, and *bad* carbohydrate.

But the sorry story does not end there. When you read the small print you will see that there are all sorts of other additives. Some are there to make the bread tasty. So you find that sweeteners have been added like corn syrup, malto-dextrin, even honey. And these are all *bad* carbohydrates.

Some additives are there as 'improvers'. What they do is improve shelf life. How do you improve shelf life? You stop bugs, bacteria and funguses from breeding in the bread. So bread often contains preservatives to kill bugs, bacteria and funguses.

What about whole-wheat bread? Surely that is all right? Almost certainly not. When you read the fine print you will very often see that in addition to the wholemeal flour, there is still the familiar "enriched" wheat flour. That is, the denatured white flour discussed above. And of course there are still the *bad* carbohydrates, fungicides and pesticides.

Why do the manufacturers go to all this trouble? Surely it would be easier simply to take the whole grain, grind it up, throw in some yeast and bake it like generations of our forefathers?

As a matter of fact, no! True whole-wheat bread is actually quite hard to make. It requires several hours for the dough to rise. The results are variable. The baking process also gives unpredictable results. It needs constant human attention to steer the process to a successful conclusion. None of these characteristics endears itself to a manufacturer who needs to have the throughput, predictability and mechanization of the production line.

That is why the nature of bread has changed so dramatically since World War II. Year by year the manufacturers have been tuning their process, denaturing and adulterating the ingredients, to give higher and higher productivity, less and less waste, more competitive pricing and tastier sales.

There is another factor: until recent times people ground their own flour immediately before baking the bread and consuming it. Part of the equipment of the Roman legionary was a hand mill. Why was this necessary? If you grind wheat into flour it only keeps for a day or two. The released oils are essential fatty acids and they go rancid in a short while.

This is a very inconvenient property of fresh flour. So today, millers take great care to treat the flour so as to eliminate or de-activate these fragile fatty acids. Result? Yet more nutrients are lost.

For these multiple reasons, bread, although it still bears the same name, is simply not the same product known to our forebears in antiquity.

What is to be done? As a Natural Eater you will be using bread frugally anyway. And when you do use it, go for the truly whole-grain bread, made only from stone ground whole-grains, yeast, and maybe a pinch of salt. If possible it will be 'whole kernel', with a high percentage (up to 50%) of the bulk being literally whole grains. not ground into flour.

Breads like this can still be found in supermarkets, often at the delicatessen counter. More often it is to be found in Health Food stores (but still read the small print), speciality bakers and outlets which carry imported German 'whole kernel rye bread'. Be prepared to find that this kind of bread is much heavier and chewy.

It is a salutary lesson that food adulteration has a long and dishonorable history. We can be sure that, from the first days that food was processed 10,000 years ago, there would be someone else who found profit in padding it out with cheap substitutes. Governments of all complexions have passed laws to protect the consumer as much as possible. For example the Germans still have a 16th Century food law controlling the ingredients for 'vollkorn brot', basic whole rye or wheat bread. It contains whole flour, yeast, salt and that's it.

3. Caffeine

A lot of confusion surrounds the use of caffeine. It is present in modest quantities in most of vegetation. Human biochemistry copes perfectly with these low doses of caffeine It is only in certain plants that the concentrations reach mind-altering proportions.

For that reason, caffeine has been investigated for many years. In relatively small quantities (100 mg/day) it can give increased mental performance and improve mood. At this dosage, the drawbacks to caffeine use are minimal. Increasing the dosage doesn't bring increased benefit and some unpleasant symptoms start to appear. Caffeine doesn't display the phenomenon of tolerance, so ever-increasing doses are not required to achieve the same effect. On the other hand, some people suffer unpleasant withdrawal symptoms when they stop taking it.

From the Natural Eating point of view, caffeine does display one drawback in some people, the raising of insulin levels. For this reason its consumption should be restricted.

Product	Quantity (for one drink)	Caffeine mg
Ground coffee	10 g (2 tsp)	180
Instant coffee	5 g (1 tsp)	50
Tea	1 teabag	50
Coca Cola	12 oz can	44
Cocoa Powder	10 g (2 tsp)	09

There is frequently a lot of confusion about the quantity of caffeine in various commonly consumed drinks. This table helps to get the position into perspective. It can be seen that ground coffee is heavily caffeinated, instant coffee, tea and the colas moderately so, and cocoa only very lightly.

4. Dietary Supplements
(Vitamins, Minerals and Other Micro-Nutrients)

Many people think that it is a good idea to take supplements, particularly if they have a medical condition. But this is a very narrow way of looking at nutrition. As explained in Chapter Eight, there are literally thousands of compounds that are important to the harmonious functioning of the body, and they all need to be working together. It is totally unrealistic to think that we can compensate for dietary errors by cherry-picking this or that supplement.

Worse, as you will have seen in Chapter Four, dosing up on one compound can have all kinds of unforeseen and detrimental ramifications. For example, taking calcium is quite useless in isolation. Your body has its own ideas about whether or not it wants to absorb the calcium from the gut, and further ideas about where to put the calcium if it is absorbed.

Dietary errors can cause your body to lay calcium down in places where it causes mischief. It crystallizes out in the kidneys as kidney stones, it clogs up the arteries as plaque and it precipitates out as painful spurs in the joints. All this because your hormones are giving the wrong instructions. Hormones do that all the time when they are upset by incorrect dietary practices, like eating too much protein, *bad* carbohydrate, or *bad* fat. Moral? You can't micro-manage – or double-guess – the complex chemical reactions going on in the body.

The central tenet of the Natural Eating concept is that all the nutrients that humans need can be, and should be, found in the foods that they eat, provided that they eat the right kinds of foods in the right patterns.

> The whole thrust of the Natural Eating message is to discourage people from the prevailing idea that they can rectify dietary errors by 'taking a pill'.

This is the ideal. However there is a small difficulty. In today's world we are all obliged to eat foods that are produced by agro-industrial methods. Plants don't always need exactly the same minerals in their feed as humans do. A hydroponically[1] grown lettuce, for example will be perfectly healthy. It has been grown using nutrients that are essential to lettuces. No one takes responsibility for ensuring that the lettuce is also being fed with the nutrients necessary for humans.

That is an extreme case. But ordinary soils too can be deficient, either by intensive farming or just because they are made that way. With the current state of farming and legislation, the consumer is not told whether the plant food he is eating has its full complement of micro-nutrients. Does it matter? For the average Westerner, that is not the first priority. Because he has such a low consumption of plant food in general, he is terribly deficient in a vast range of micro-nutrients. Indeed, it is quipped that our populations suffer from 'affluenza', malnutrition in the midst of plenty.

Consequence? Take just one example, the immune system.

Micro-nutrients, although needed in minute quantities, form an indispensable link in a chain of chemical reactions supporting the immune system. And our immune systems are vitally important in keeping us alive. Our bodies are a daily battleground between our immune system and a vast array of enemies that want to overrun it.

—————— ◆ ——————

Our bodies are a battleground between our immune system and a vast array of enemies.

—————— ◆ ——————

These enemies are bacteria, viruses and other external parasites. More insidiously, there also is an enemy within. We know that cells are going cancerous in their thousands every minute, and that rogue cells and toxic products are being created the whole time from sunlight, from what we eat, even from parasitical genes in our DNA. Our immune system never sleeps and is ever vigilant. It tirelessly patrols our bodies seeking out and destroying enemy agents.

---

1 Many plants, like tomatoes and lettuces are grown intensively without any soil at all. Their roots just hang in water laced with the necessary nutrients for that plant. This is known as hydroponic cultivation.

At least, ideally it is. The trouble with the way we eat today is that the foot patrols are sluggish from malnourishment. To be alert and vigorous, they need feeding with a liberal supply of micronutrients and antioxidants. Yes, you know the answer. The micro-nutrient-dense plant foods.

What about the Natural Eater who is already consuming colored plant material in large quantities? What is the likelihood that he is suffering any deficiencies? The answer is, "unlikely." With the remarkable modern network of food supply and distribution, we are receiving fruits, salads and vegetables cultivated on a huge variety of agricultural territories all around the world. Vary the food types and vary their origins and you will surely avoid any particular deficiency.

Even so, many people like the reassurance of understanding the micro-nutrients most at risk of deficiency. Even the best eating pattern in today's world can only be as good as the products that are made available. It is legitimate, where all else fails, and however imperfect that might be, to make good possible shortfalls with supplements. The list of at-risk micro-nutrients is very short. The nature of these vitamins and minerals and their sub-RDA[2] top-up dosage is discussed at greater length in the Natural Eating Manual.

5. Organic Foods

Let's say straight up front that the organic food movement is a worthy one and deserves every support and encouragement. It is certainly in the health interests of all consumers to roll back the excesses of agro-industrial production methods. The wanton use of pesticides and chemicals of all kinds serves only one purpose: the production of quantity without regard to nutritional quality, pollution or long term population health. The violence that is done to the environment is very worrying, and in the long run unsustainable. Beautiful landscape is reduced to a moonscape in the interests of mechanical efficiency. Agro-industry is in a never-ending arms race with insects that become resistant, a plant gene pool that is ever more effete and soils that are exhausted and depleted.

In a time when farmers are now being paid to not grow crops, a major change in direction is possible. We now have the luxury of being able to backtrack. To trade off lower yields for a gentler farming regime. We can use all the arts of organic farming to get a reasonable return out of a farming process that works in harmony with the environment and still feed us all. For this to happen, consumers will have to change too. In particular, be prepared to pay a little more. Buy organic and eschew the technicolor perfection of supermarket produce.

Now to answer the question! What are the priorities? Is eating organic the main priority when seeking good nutrition? Not necessarily! Just think, does a smoker worry if his tobacco is organic. Of course not. The main

2 RDA. Recommended Daily Amount.

problem is the tobacco itself.

There are many foods that are just as dangerous whether or not they are organic. Thus organic sugar, organic bread, organic butter, and organic pork are all just as bad as the regular sort.

We have to look beyond the simple label 'organic' to find a deeper truth. One of the greatest dietary errors in the West is the low consumption of plant food. The adverse health consequences are grave and measurable. The adverse health consequences of eating agro-industrial foods are much smaller. Therefore, the highest priority is to eat more plant food from whatever source. Eating 'organic' is good, but a second order of priority.

6. Sweeteners

Human beings have a sweet tooth. This betrays our origins as a frugivore[3]. We still retain the programming to seek out our ancient naturally adapted food, fruits. Yet this is a double edged sword (or a blunt instrument). Our instincts are undiscriminating. Sweetness per se is all we seek. The genius of food technology today has removed the link between sweetness and wholesome food.

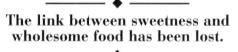

The link between sweetness and wholesome food has been lost.

Human ingenuity has developed sources of sweetness that have absolutely no place in our genetic programming. Most notably this is from sugar cane and sugar beet. Sugar cane originated in Southeast Asia and was known to the Indian civilization several thousand years ago. At that time the cane was chewed whole.

Alexander the Great, in his conquest of the Ganges area during the 3rd Century B.C., reported the existence of a "stiff grass yielding a kind of honey." This was the first contact of Western civilizations with primitive sugar cane. Even so, it was not until the long voyages of European exploration that crude sugar refining was invented and sugar itself became a trading commodity.

Only the aristocracy could afford it. Famously, Elizabeth I received presents of loaf sugar from the king of Morocco. Famously too, Elizabeth suffered excruciatingly from a mouthful of rotten teeth.

It was not until the development of sugar plantations in tropical America during the 18th Century that sugar became commonly available. (Remember the graph of sugar consumption in Chapter Four?)

As for beet sugar, this is an even more recent development. Germany was cut off from the lucrative sugar trade dominated by Spanish, Portuguese

---

3 Fruit eating creature. Also known as 'fructivore'.

and British interests. Their scientists devised methods of extracting sugar from beets. They succeeded very well, and today over half the world's sugar production comes from sugar beet.

These are very recent developments, really in the last two centuries. And there is a problem. This type of sugar 'common sugar' is known as sucrose. As explained in Chapter Four, not only are we consuming large quantities of this sugar, our bodies bio-chemistry is ill adapted to it. It is making us sick.

Common sugar is a disaccharide, which means that its molecule has two components. In sucrose one molecule is glucose and the other is fructose. Glucose is the harmful one. It gets digested directly into the bloodstream very fast, causing those dangerous insulin peaks.

Fructose (the sweet tasting element in most fruit) has to go to the liver first to be converted to glucose. As a result, it enters the bloodstream slowly and at a controlled rate. Insulin is secreted in normal quantities. Fructose is the harmless one, it is the sugar to which we are naturally adapted.

Fructose taken alone has a low glycemic index (G.I.) of 20. Sugar, having a 50% glucose component, has a dangerously high G.I. of 65. Most fruits therefore have a low G.I. But be wary. Check the schedules in Appendix 1. We do not eat a single fruit today that would be recognized by our African Pleistocene ancestors. All the fruits that we eat today have been cultivated and developed from primitive stocks from almost everywhere in the world except the East African savannah. Furthermore, many fruits, such as the melon and the grape have been bred down the millennia to increase their sweetness. No one was paying attention at the time as to whether this sweetness came from sucrose or fructose.

Is fructose a free-lunch? Not entirely. Even the large daily ration of two pounds of fruit does not contain more than a couple of tablespoons of fructose, whereas the average daily consumption of sugar in the US is one-half pound. If we were to make a simple substitution of fructose for sugar in the average Western diet, there would be other drawbacks.

First, fructose is still empty calories, fattening and no nutrients. Second, high fructose levels raise triglycerides and cholesterol levels. Finally, fructose in abnormal quantities can cause gastro-intestinal upsets.

So is there a place for fructose in the Natural Eating Pattern? Yes, it can still serve as a sweetener in the occasional dessert, such as the chocolate gateau recipe given in Chapter Twelve. Otherwise go very easy on it.

Also don't be misled either by 'high fructose corn syrup[4]'. It is still at least 50% glucose and has just the same bad G.I. as sugar itself. As for the other sugar aliases, malto-dextrin, dextrose, malt, maltose and indeed glucose itself, they are all bad sugars.

---

4 High fructose corn syrup is a very common ingredient in processed foods, soft drinks etc. as can be readily seen on the ingredient lists. Just read 'sugar' when you see 'high fructose corn syrup'.

What about other 'natural' sweeteners like honey and maple syrup? After all honey holds a venerable position in civilized cuisine down the centuries. It is true that the art of bee-keeping was developed during classical times, but the amounts of honey available were always modest and were restricted to the upper classes. Regrettably, honey and maple syrup are mostly sucrose too, and are just as bad for health. Honey is fine for bees' bio-chemistry; not so good for a human's.

Finally what about artificial sweeteners?

From a purist point of view, Aspartame, saccharine and the like, never formed part of the Pleistocene diet. Nevertheless, they have been exhaustively tested. If sugar had been obliged to pass the same regulations as artificial sweeteners, it would have been banned as a dangerous substance. Recent studies suggest that up to 150,000 premature deaths a year in America can be attributed to the consumption of sugar!

Just imagine the outcry if *just one death* could be attributed to the use of an artificial sweetener. In a world where we sometimes have to choose the lesser of two evils then, as a first step, substituting Aspartame (say) for sugar, is very definitely a move in the right direction.

———— ◆ ————

Substitution of an artificial sweetener for sugar is the lesser of two evils.

———— ◆ ————

There is another class of bulk artificial sweeteners, the 'sugar alcohols' such as sorbitol, maltitol and the like. They have very low glycemic indexes, but like fructose, should not be abused either. They are less sweet and have a very pronounced laxative effect. The authorities still haven't got consensus on their safe and appropriate utilization.

7. Pesticides

Man is a species that is designed to live on the fringes of the tropical rain forests. For thousands of generations our ancestors browsed for their food. That is, they lived off the land eating what was available in the environment around them.

When you live like this, a large territory is required to be sure of always having enough to eat, some 8 sq. miles per person. Today, even an empty country like the United States has a density of 80 *people* per square mile. Western Europe is even more densely populated, with over 300 people per square mile.

Plainly, we are well beyond the point of no return. There is no going back to our Pleistocene foraging patterns. The hard truth is that we can only feed our populations by farming methods. And as the populations increase, so farming methods get more *intensive*.

Does this matter? Many people get worried particularly about the use of pesticides.

Today our food chain relies heavily on the use of agro-chemicals. That is the penalty of having a population that far exceeds our naturally adapted population density.

People often ask "Won't I be eating a lot of pesticides by consuming more fruit and vegetables?" The reality is that pesticides get into everything we eat – bread, cereals, meat, fish, milk and, yes, fruits and vegetables.

The good news is that the body has ways of eliminating most of these pollutants, on condition that the organs of elimination – chiefly, the liver, kidneys and intestine are not overloaded by poor eating habits.

It may come as a surprise to know that pesticides are naturally present in all vegetation. Many insects enjoy eating plants, and the plants on the whole don't like it. Over the eons during which plants and insects have coexisted, plants have developed a battery of insect poisons, or 'pesticides'. Many modern pesticides are developed from these natural plant pesticides.

The good news is that the human body is well adapted to coping with many plant pesticides. Human beings have evolved over long periods of time as plant eaters to the point where our body chemistry has got very good at dealing with pesticides.

Consider too, that foodstuffs are regularly tested by the regulatory authorities for pesticides. In the large majority of cases no measurable quantity is detected. In a minority of samples there are measurable quantities but, in view of the wide safety factors built into the benchmarks, still within the safe limits.

What can the ordinary consumer do to limit his exposure? Note that the alleged ill effects of consuming pesticides in food are still largely speculative. On the other hand the ill effects of eating foods polluted by bacteria are proven, and cases of food poisoning occur all the time.

Cleaning up bacteria is a much more important priority than going after pesticides. How do you do that? By washing the produce in soapy water. There are proprietary fruit and vegetable 'surfactants' sold in good supermarkets and health food stores. Even ordinary washing liquid is effective. Either way, give the produce a good rinse afterwards.

Remember, only 1% of the fruit or vegetables are likely to have any trace of pesticide anyway. What you will be washing off is bacteria and the wax coating that is put on to preserve freshness.

Much more problematic is meat. You shouldn't be eating much of it, but if you do, cut off the visible fat. That can reduce the pesticide content by up to two-thirds, and it does your fat-intake profile some good into the bargain.

Worse, is the latent contamination from bacteria like E-coli and salmonella. These can't be washed off. Thorough cooking is the answer. If you are eating cold meats like ham and meat pâté, then you are really vulnerable. First take care not to cross contaminate from raw meat, and second, cross your fingers that the food manufacture had high standards of cleanliness.

Back to pesticides. Think of this, if your cat has a flea collar, or you use insecticide sprays in the home, then you are probably exposed to more pesticide than you are ever likely to get in your diet. It is too easy to get anxious about insecticide in the food supply whilst remaining quite insouciant about zapping that bluebottle with an aerosol.

The bottom line? We are designed as plant-eating creatures. You will certainly do yourself a big favor by eating naturally. Consume large quantities of fruits, vegetables and salads. Get that right and the body will take care of the rest.

8. Salt (Sodium Chloride)

Yes, we all eat it to excess, and it matters. Don't allow your critical faculties to be dulled by the conflicting messages over the salt/blood pressure connection. Does high salt consumption increase blood pressure? It all depends who you listen to. Some people are salt sensitive, and their blood pressure shows a clear increase with increased salt consumption. Others do not show this relationship.

But this is not the point. As described in Chapter Three, our naturally adapted diet was low in salt and particularly the salt/potassium ratio was low. Today, that situation is reversed and the health consequences are multiple. Blood pressure is only one factor that can be affected.

High sodium levels affect calcium metabolism. Over-consumption of salt drains calcium out of the bones. This is just one more example of how today's dietary practices are greasing the slippery slope towards osteoporosis.

Excess salt scars arteries. We tend to think of our arteries as being a bit like inert plastic piping. In reality they are living tissue, they react to what is passing through them. High salt levels irritate and scar the arteries – one more factor in the development of atherosclerosis.

Finally, the body is constantly having to battle the imbalance in the salt/potassium ratio. The kidneys are put under stress and in the worst outcome they fail altogether.

Is there any relief from this scenario? Yes there is, the high consumption of fruits can mitigate markedly these effects. You don't have to drive salt out of your life altogether. A vast improvement can be achieved by reducing salt somewhat and increasing plant food greatly.

The biggest enemy is salt in processed food. It was brought home to me forcefully when, many years ago, I was involved with a salt project in the Hauts Plateaux of North Africa. The factory was to extract salt from a deep underground stratum by injecting steam down one borehole and recovering brine from an adjacent bore-hole. 30,000 tons per year were planned to be extracted. This seemed to me an enormous quantity and I assumed the salt would be used as feedstock for the manufacture of some other bulk chemical.

None of it! Imagine my astonishment when I was told that all this salt, 30,000 tons per year, were to be shipped to a pea canning factory. It was a powerful lesson. Almost every processed product has a strong dose of salt.

Why do manufacturers use all this salt? Regrettably the consumer is partly to blame; he likes the taste. There is a more sinister reason too. It is well known that salted nibbles are supplied in bars. They make the customers thirsty so that they drink more. What is happening? Your kidneys have to get rid of this excess salt, so they draw fluid out of the body to do it.

"Fear Greeks bearing gifts." The free nibble is the bar owner's invitation to disrupt your salt/potassium ratio and put your body under dehydration stress. This lesson has not been lost on the soft drink manufacturers either. Almost every soft drink contains its gratuitous quota of salt. A can of Sprite has over 50 mg of salt.

Salt has other tasty properties too. For example, it helps processed foods retain water. Salt is used for bulking. Ham manufacturers save on pork by injecting it with water – up to 20% of the weight. The trouble is this water has an irritating tendency to leak out. By injecting the ham with salt the water stays in place. Imagine the satisfaction of the manufacturers. They succeed in selling you a product that is 20% injected water and you don't even mind because it has a nice salty taste too!

These are just some examples of how salt is used in processed foods. Everything to do with profitable sales and nothing to do with the nutritional health of the consumer.

Be savvy when looking for the salt taste. How many of you enjoy the salty taste of cornflakes? Most people don't realize that cornflakes have more salt than seawater! Or that salted peanuts have *less* salt than cornflakes. The salt in cornflakes and many other processed products is gratuitous. You can't taste it but, unnoticed, it is adding significantly to your salt imbalances. Look out for the sodium on the food labels. Avoid gratuitous salt.

Lesson: Salt added to the outside of the food is much more noticeable than if it is processed into the food. Get the most taste for the least salt. Add the salt (if you have to) onto the food just before you eat it.

———— ◆ ————

Added salt is much more noticeable than salt processed in.

———— ◆ ————

Are salt substitutes any better than salt itself? Most salt substitutes are based on potassium chloride. (Salt is sodium chloride.) Potassium and sodium are very similar metals and their salts have similar properties, and that includes taste.

However, in the body their action is rather different. Potassium, which is plentiful in fruits, is an important 'antidote' to salt.

The short answer is that a salt substitute has the potential to be an improvement on table salt. However, there is a catch. If potassium is consumed in the same vast quantities that people absorb table salt, then there are big draw-backs. Potassium chloride in mega-doses also damages kidneys and other organs.

The message is, reduce salt of all kinds. With that proviso, the use of modest amounts of salt substitute is fine.

9. Nutritional Profile of the Natural Eating Pattern

Right up till now, we have mentioned little about how the nutritional content of the Natural Eating Pattern measures against conventional orthodox wisdom. This is deliberate. Our Pleistocene ancestors managed very well for over a million years and they didn't give the question a single thought.

Think of it, every one of us alive today is descended from succeeding generations of fathers and mothers in an unbroken chain, who successfully conceived, raised and brought to puberty at least one offspring. Not one of them failed! Every one of our ancestors back into the dawn of time was healthy and strong enough to do that. And they never counted calcium, calories or cholesterol.

Nevertheless, we do live in an age when we are aware of such things, so it is unrealistic to think that this question should not be addressed.

Dozens of typical days have been analyzed for nutritional content as part of the Natural Eating Pattern. Breakdowns of a typical day's eating have been made for the major food groups (fat, protein, etc.), all the major vitamins and their groups and a very broad range of micro-nutrients. The results are uniformly remarkable. On all measures, the diet furnishes supremely healthy amounts of good nutrients. Moreover, these come in the right combinations and proportions. Harmful constituents are attenuated to healthy levels.

It is reassuring, but not surprising, to know that eating naturally provides all the nutrients recommended by conventional calculations.

———— ◆ ————

Natural Eating provides all the nutrients recommended by conventional norms

———— ◆ ————

In this connection it is pertinent to explore certain features of 'conventional' calculations and to point up their limitations:

* Recommended Daily Allowances (RDA's) for many nutrients have been established by most national authorities. In the United States they are now known as Recommended Nutritional Intakes (R.N.I.). They have their limitations, for example:

The RDA for vitamin C is 75 mg./day for women and 90 mg./day for men. This is the minimum to stop you getting scurvy. For optimum health you need at least 5 times as much.

Calcium is set high, simply because of our other dietary errors, but still does not address the fundamental problem of what the body does with it.

* RDAs are set as 'one size fits all'. That is, the quantity that will cover every citizen (in the U.S. 97% of all citizens), whether male or female, whatever weight or size, whatever age and whatever their genetic inheritance or real need. A figure is then decided for the most extreme case and then this figure is multiplied by a safety factor. For the average person, the RDA can be as much as three times what they really need. This is completely at odds with the idea that micro-nutrients interact with each other in quite unpredictable ways. Like vitamin C and calcium above, they can be way off because we don't understand, let alone control, all the ramifications of a complete nutrient intake.

* RDAs have not been established for many micro-nutrients such as chromium, boron and vanadium, to say nothing of the tens of thousands of phytochemicals such as bioflavonoids, terpenes, phenols and carotenoids (see Chapter Eight). The only way to be sure of getting these micro-nutrients in the right proportions and combinations is to eat the natural foodstuff in which they are packaged.

———— ◆ ————

Eating naturally is the only sure way of getting the full complement of nutrients that the body needs.

———— ◆ ————

Finally, the regulatory authorities are slowly coming to the view that it is possible to have too much of a good thing. Remember again those 'networks' in Chapter Four? Too much copper can deplete zinc for example? Even this seemingly trivial question can have serious consequences. Studies[5] have shown that young men become more violent if they have unbalanced copper/zinc ratios. Yet one more example of the law of unintended consequences.

The authorities have become conscious of this danger, that more of a good thing does not necessarily mean better. Bodies like the Institute of Medicine (IOM), have a committee wrestling with setting safe *maximum* intakes for key nutrients.

But you do not have to wait on their ponderous deliberations. Just eat naturally and the quantities will just work out fine.

10. Lifespan in Historical Times

There is a prevalent illusion that we live longer and better than people in historical times. This is perhaps driven by our images of life in the fetid cities so graphically described by Charles Dickens and Victor Hugo. Sure, in those days, and in those places, life was indeed "mean, nasty, brutish and short" for many people. But that is hardly a standard by which we should judge our prosperous and pampered lives today. The reality is that rural Americans have much the same life expectancy at 15 as did their great grandparents 150 years ago.

What about the prosperous and pampered societies further back in time? It is a central thesis of this book that neither the lifestyle of ancient agricultural civilizations nor those of Medieval and Victorian Europe are a good model for us today. Nevertheless, it helps to cast the spotlight on a number of issues.

After the farming revolution 10,000 years ago, for the first time in the history of the human race, people were living in close proximity with each other and they were dependent on farming. For the first time, human populations were exposed to the hazards of crop failure, new diseases – particularly new diseases – and disastrous floods and plagues.

Babies were born at more frequent intervals, but more babies died in infancy. This drags down the averages. After a natural disaster whole populations would be wiped out. The technology of warfare became ever more murderous. But how are we to put on a statistically sound basis a true estimate of longevity? The answer is that we cannot.

To get another bearing on the question, we can look at what the ancient peoples themselves thought of their life expectancy.

First, a quick look at the writings of the ancient Greek, Homer. Based on Homer's directions in the Iliad, the archeologist Schlieman discovered the site of Homer's 3,000 year old Troy in 1870. It was a dramatic vindication of the historical basis of Homer's stories about Odysseus. Homer relates

5 Walsh et al; Copper and Zinc Levels Influence Behavior; Physiology & Behavior; 1997; 1(8)

how Odysseus' wife Penelope remained faithful even though he was absent for twenty years. The remarkable, but little commented feature is that Penelope was besieged by ardent suitors for the twenty years of Odysseus' absence. Some of the suitors were the same age as her son Telemachus.

In other words, in ancient Greece, 3,000 years ago, a 40-plus woman was such a marriageable attraction that she was pursued by men half her age!

Around about the same time, three thousand years ago, the writer of Psalm 90 was saying "the days of our years are three score years and ten; and if by reason of strength they be four score years, yet is their strength labor and sorrow; for it is soon cut off and we fly away."

In other words, 3,000 years ago, in the biblical late Bronze Age, it was thought normal to live to at least 70 years old, and with a bit of good health to 80.

Or we can look at the words of Aristotle living in ancient Greece over 2,300 years ago. He recommended that men wait until they are 35 years old before even getting married. The Greeks in general thought that a man reached his peak at the age of 40. These are hardly the strategies of people expecting a short life or a decrepit old age.

Look again at some of Alexander the Great's generals. Antigonus Monophthalmos was a battling veteran who, encouraging his troops from his war-horse, finally succumbed to a hail of javelins at the Battle of Ipsus. He was 81 years old. His opponent, Lysimichos was later killed at the Battle of Coropedium at the age of 79. His ally Selfcos Nicator survived all battles only to be assassinated at the age of 78.

This is the other side of the coin, old men with a youth's vigor. Old men who could lead their troops into battle, wielding the heavy armament of the period.

———— ◆ ————

Ancient Greeks carried youth into old age.

———— ◆ ————

Of course, this is all just circumstantial evidence. Yet it is surely no coincidence that the ancient Greek diet is still represented, 23 centuries later, by the much studied, and healthful, Cretan diet discussed in Chapter Three.

C h a p t e r   E i g h t

The Food/Disease Connection

Most, if not all, of the so-called 'diseases of civilization' are quite avoidable. Many that have become entrenched can be cured or ameliorated. In all of them, our eating patterns are the major factor, although often other lifestyle factors play a role too.

Not surprisingly, eating naturally is most likely to give you the best chance of improvement. By eating naturally you are removing the factors from the diet that are causing distress to your body biochemistry. You are eating in harmony with the way your body is designed.

In Chapter Two, *The Rewards*, we looked at some of the maladies that find relief in eating naturally. In this chapter we shall look at just what exactly can make the difference in each case.

All the recommendations are supported by a plethora of scientific studies: clinical trials, epidemiological studies, anthropological studies (studies on primitive peoples) and of course our understanding of how our Pleistocene ancestors adapted to their food supply.

Not surprisingly, the reader will note that there are common factors too. These all go to reinforce the notion that eating naturally really is the only sensible way to go.

Scientifically, there is still enormous ignorance about what different foodstuffs contain. It's a theme that we come back to frequently in this book. By clinical trials and population trials, we are zeroing in on the foods that are helpful, without always being able to explain why.

We know that there are literally tens of thousands of active compounds in the foods we eat, particularly fruits and vegetables. We can't define exactly how all these compounds work, but we ignore their importance at our peril.

For example, a tremendous amount of damage is done in the body by free radicals. Free radicals are molecules charging about, looking to unite with another molecule and oxidize it. If the target molecule is in a vital part of the body, its function is destroyed or perverted. Our bodies are designed to work with a variety of anti-oxidants. These are molecules which scavenge the free radicals and neutralize them.

> *Note that the guide lines given in this chapter are not intended to replace or supplant the advice of your medical practitioner. If you have a medical disorder, you should first see your doctor.*

Where are anti-oxidants found? Almost exclusively in fruits and vegetation. There are literally thousands of anti-oxidants and only in a very few instances do we fully understand how they operate. The more well known ones are vitamin C, vitamin E, zinc and selenium.

There are also the carotenoids, of which there are over 600. They give the colour for example to carrots, oranges, tomatoes and melons.

Then there are the 5,000 phenol compounds. They too are present in all fruits and vegetables. They are strongly present in tea, coffee and wine.

And again, there are the 7,000 terpene compounds. Terpenes too are omnipresent in all plant foods. They are particularly present in all kinds of spices and aromatic herbs. The terpenes appear to have a particularly strong suppressive effect on cancer cells, even to the point of causing them to behave like normal cells again.

We must not forget the thousands of bioflavonoids, yet another vast range of compounds that are essential to the body. We know that they are important to optimum health, and the only way to be sure of getting them, is by eating plant foods.

Note that supplements are not the solution: what supplement contains the 5,000 phenols, the 7,000 terpenes, the 600 carotenoids, the thousands of bioflavonoids, the dozens of trace minerals and the essential vitamins? There's only one place they all come together neatly packaged – in fruits and vegetables!

So the message is: For optimum health 'eat naturally'. That way you are sure of harmonizing your intake of nutrients to the needs of your body. Today of course, hardly anyone eats this way and as a result the population is suffering various 'deficiency diseases'.

The 'diseases of civilization' are deficiency diseases.

There is a huge variation in people's genetic make-up and in their ability to circumvent deficiencies in the diet. That is why, even though eating the same way, different people will develop different illnesses.

The rest of this chapter is devoted to setting out our current knowledge of what foods are helpful and what foods are not helpful for specific illnesses and what we should do about it. If you suffer from any of these conditions, then you will do well to concentrate, in the first instance, on the recommendations specific to that condition.

Nevertheless, when all the recommendations are put together, you will see that they converge on the Golden Rules for Natural Eating. So why take a chance? Think about going the whole hog straight away.

Rheumatoid Arthritis, Osteo-Arthritis, Multiple Sclerosis, Lupus

These diseases are made more difficult because their causes are often multiple: a malfunctioning immune system, allergic reaction or a deficiency in the diet of essential nutrients. Diet is not always going to be the main culprit, but getting the diet right will stack the cards in favour of resolving the condition.

Arthritis has been linked to a deficiency of antioxidants. Yes, plant foods again. Many studies show that arthritis sufferers have a history of low consumption of fruits, and vegetables, and that they have abnormally low blood levels of anti-oxidants like vitamins C and E and beta-carotene. There are certainly many other compounds in fruits and vegetables (read the first few paragraphs of this chapter) that are essential too. The first priority of an arthritis sufferer is to boost dramatically his intake of plant food.

The second culprit is the overproduction of inflammatory chemicals induced particularly by 'Omega 6' oils. These oils are complete novelties to the human diet, having become common only since World War II. In the body, Omega 6 oils are transformed into all kinds of chemical messengers. Some of these are histamines and leukotrienes. These are substances that instruct cells to inflame, swell and secrete mucus. So the second big priority is to cut out Omega 6 oils.

A third culprit is saturated fat in all its forms: animal origin, plant origin and man-made (margarines, trans-fatty acids and hydrogenated fats). Saturated fats block and interrupt the work of helpful chemical messengers. It is essential to follow Natural Eating principles in this matter and ruthlessly cut out saturated fats.

The counterpart to that is to consume some 'Omega 3' oils. These are transformed in the body into chemical messengers that do the opposite to 'Omega 6', by instructing cells to stop inflaming, secreting mucus and swelling. So it is a high priority to consume modestly Omega 3 oils. This action must be accompanied by a ruthless reduction in the *bad* fats (Omega 6 oils, saturated fats, hydrogenated fats and trans-fatty acids.)

Oily fish contain similar compounds to Omega 3 oils and so are also recommended.

Finally, arthritis is often triggered by an allergic reaction. Some of the commonest allergens are foods that humans were never designed to eat: wheat, corn and dairy products. Refer also to the segment on allergies later in this chapter.

Multiple Sclerosis and Lupus: These are diseases that remain largely a mystery to medical science. However, studies show that at least two factors are implicated, a dysfunctional fatty acid metabolism and low levels of blood anti-oxidants. Starts to sound familiar?

If you suffer from one of these conditions you will certainly stack the deck of cards in your favour if you adopt the Natural Eating precepts. Lay particular emphasis on the "helpful foods". Read the segment later in this chapter that deals with auto-immune diseases.

For Food/Arthritis summary see p. 156.

Cardiovascular Diseases

Heart Disease, Atherosclerosis, Thrombosis, Strokes, High Blood Pressure, High Cholesterol

These diseases are stereotypical of modern civilization. They are unknown amongst the primitive tribes, like the Australian Aborigines, the Tarahumaras, the Hunzas and even the Eskimos. As far as we can tell, they were unknown amongst our Pleistocene forebears. What is at the root of these illnesses? The main problem is to do with the disturbing of hormonal balances. Particularly hormones like insulin, thrombin and adrenaline. When these hormones are floating around in the bloodstream in abnormal quantities, they create mischief. What do they do? They act on the walls of the blood vessels in many ways, with the net result of causing the production of plaque and blood clots.

Referring back to Chapter Five, the main culprits are the *bad* carbohydrates and the *bad* fats. They are quite unnatural foods for humans to be eating and, as luck would have it, they do have an extremely deleterious effect on human biochemistry.

How reversible are these diseases? That depends. The main objective has to be to stop the rot. The risks of strokes and thrombosis can be quickly reduced by changing dietary habits. Thromboxane, the hormone chiefly implicated, is reduced almost overnight by cutting *bad* fats. High blood pressure is brought down to a greater or lesser degree over a few months. Reversing arterial damage is more problematic. Here the emphasis has to be on stopping further deterioration.

The story on artery damage is not yet finished. Where proteins come from is also significant. Animal protein has a strongly atherogenic (artery damaging) effect, and milk proteins (casein) are the worst. Therefore these are to be reduced. And plant proteins? Yet another straw in the wind. Plant proteins are helpful to the artery walls.

So, the main strategy is to eliminate *bad* carbohydrates, animal proteins and *bad* fats from the diet and stop further corrosion of the cardiovascular

Tip: People who live in hard water areas have lower levels of arterial disease. The more your water pipes fur up, the less your arteries fur up.

It seems that calcium is best absorbed in small quantities drip-fed in throughout the day. Calcium absorbed this way is artery helpful.

system. Just by doing that, the body can start to repair some of the damage.

The task of repairing the damage is accelerated if the body has correct supplies of nutrients. This is where fruits, salads and vegetables come in. Remember at the start of this chapter there was information about anti-oxidants? We particularly need these to stop free radicals damaging the walls of the arteries. Furthermore, plant foods together with their fibre get the body's cardiovascular hormones functioning in harmony.

So much for arteries, thromboses and strokes. What about high blood pressure? Contrary to popular wisdom, salt is not always a culprit. However, salt does damage the arteries, so it is best avoided. High blood pressure yields well to a high plant-food diet. Here we go again. Studies, such as the 'DASH' study[1] demonstrate that a diet high in fruits and vegetables significantly reduces blood pressure.

And what do studies of the long-lived, healthy races of the world show? Studies on tribes such as the Vincambamba of the Andes and the Tarahumara of Mexico show that these peoples have low blood pressures, low cholesterol and extremely low incidence of cardio-vascular disease.

Rarely do their blood pressures exceed 130/75, *even amongst centenarians.* And these peoples have 13 times the rate of centenarians as America.

How do these peoples live? Plenty of physical activity, and a diet very close to the Natural Eating Pattern. They eat plenty of plant food, eat little or no meat and little or no milk.

For Food/CVD summary see p. 157.

The Immune System

Cancer & Auto-Immune Diseases (allergies, migraine, asthma etc..)

Cancer

We are all walking around with pre-cancerous cells in us. The only reason that they are not expressed is because our immune system is keeping the lid tightly closed on them. Even when they are expressed, sometimes a dramatic regression of the cancer can be achieved by getting the immune system up to speed, and by not undermining it with unnecessary tasks.

Cancer is a modern disease. Remarkably, for all the tens of thousands of mummified ancient Egyptian bodies studied, no sign of cancer has been found. The same is true when we look at peoples who live in the traditional primitive way. Why should this be? Why should cancer be a disease of modern industrial societies?

1 Appel L J et al; 'DASH' Study - Dietary Effect on Blood Pressure; NEJM; 1997;336;1117-24. See bibliography.

We can be fairly sure that the primary reason is the way we eat. Added to that are certain lifestyle factors like smoking, obesity, lack of exercise, and alcohol.

All the research shows that a diet that is high in plant foods is the best protection against cancer. For the Natural Eater, the reason is simple – our bodies were designed to work that way. Nevertheless, scientifically, we like to know the detail of how and why. We know that the antioxidants and other phyto-chemicals are important. But they are only effective if eaten as plant food, and not when taken as supplements. It is clear that there are many more essential compounds in plant food that we still don't know about. We do know that they all need to be present *together* to be effective.

Here are two examples of some clinical studies:

Researchers at Johns Hopkins University, in the United States have confirmed that sulphurophane blocks cancer growth. It is found concentrated in broccoli sprouts[2], and in good quantities in broccoli and other cruciferous vegetables such as cabbage, cauliflower and brussels sprouts.

Harvard University researchers find that the carotenoid lycopene, found particularly in tomatoes, protects against prostate cancer. Other research shows that allocins found in onions and garlic are protective against cancer.

Another helpful practice is to avoid saturated fats and Omega 6 oils. They depress the immune system. On the other hand, studies show that an adequate supply of the essential fatty acid, alpha linolenic acid Omega 3 oil, (vitamin F_2) reinforces the immune system and is protective for cancer.

In fact, a low fat diet is a prerequisite for a healthy anticancer diet.

———— ◆ ————

The anticancer diet is high in fruits and vegetables and low in fat.

———— ◆ ————

Other habits to avoid are fried foods and char-broiled meats. The compounds formed from the burnt fats are thought to be carcinogenic.

What about breast cancer? Everything said about cancer in general applies to breast cancer in particular. Nevertheless, there are some special remarks to be made.

Remember the saying that 'we are what we eat'? A woman's breasts furnish a good example. A woman who eats a lot of saturated fats and trans-fatty acids (hydrogenated fats) has more of those *bad* fats stored in her breasts. Such women are at much higher risk of developing breast cancer. Cut out the *bad* fats, margarines, milk, etc.

2 Broccoli sprouts are the sprouted seeds of broccoli. They look like bean sprouts or alfalfa sprouts.

Next, let's consider the insulin connection. High insulin levels increase the number of estrogen receptors in the breast by a factor of 12. This is a formula for increased tumor growth and proliferation. Moral? Keep insulin levels within normal limits, avoid the *bad* carbohydrates.

Finally, the anthropological connection. Breast cancer is practically unknown outside the West. You don't even have to clamber over the Himalayas or the Andes to find peoples who live breast cancer-free. Take a comfortable plane to Tokyo, Singapore or Hong Kong and you will immediately be amongst peoples who live longer than Westerners do, and whose women do not suffer from breast cancer. Their secret? They eat very little meat, and no milk, butter, cheese or yogurt. *They have very low fat diets.*

Infectious Disease

Having a finely tuned immune system means that you are much more resistant to infectious disease. Vulnerability to colds, flu, viruses, even food poisoning is greatly reduced.

Modern industrial human beings do not have good resistance to communicable diseases. The slightest whiff of gamy meat and they are sick. This is the phenomenon of 'affluent malnutrition'. They eat lots, but their immune systems are still deficient in certain essential elements.

Outbreaks of E-coli in Scotland, for example, killed many people. It is speculated that the Scottish immune systems are depressed due to a lack of selenium, an important anti-oxidant. Meanwhile the Eskimo prefers his caribou (and his fish) well putrefied.

Auto-immune diseases: Allergies, Migraine and Asthma

There is usually a cocktail of causes for these diseases, and the whole story is far from complete. However, there are certain dietary habits that are known to be helpful, and others that are known to be harmful. If you suffer from one of these diseases, it makes sense to eliminate at least one possible cause, the one due to harmful diet.

Allergies, migraine and asthma have many triggers. Usually the sufferer is sensitive to quite a few allergens and the allergy only breaks out when several of them have cumulated. Then it is the last one that gets the blame. Even worse, often the reaction can be delayed up to 24 hours after exposure. The average sufferer has no way of making the link between the trigger and the onset of the allergic reaction. That is why it is difficult to isolate the culprit; there are many of them and the exposure from day to day will be in a different order.

Many foods, including cheese, peanuts, pork, citrus fruits, and alcohol contain compounds called 'vasoactive amines'. These chemicals are

> **Migraine: some triggers:**
>
> - *caffeine*
> - *tyramine*
> - *monosodium glutamate*
> - *nitrates*
> - *phenols*
> - *hormonal fluctuations*
> - *weather changes*
> - *medications*
> - *stress*

related to the neurotransmitters serotonin and norepinephrine, chemical messengers in the brain, and have long been suspected of triggering migraines.

One of the meanest allergens is the medication that one takes to relieve it. Particularly with migraines, the sufferer has to start by cutting out the pain relievers. This can be tough, the process is akin to going 'cold turkey' from an addictive drug. But it has to be the starting point in the search for a migraine management strategy.

In any allergic condition, it may be necessary to go squarely onto an 'elimination diet'. Fast for 24 hours on water and then gradually introduce a new foodstuff day by day. Sticking to the strict Natural Eating diet should make this easier. It is not surprising that the commonest allergens are the foods that are foreign novelties for the human race, like wheat and dairy products – the very products that should be the first to be eliminated by any practitioner of Natural Eating.

One major disrupter are the cereal lectins. These are the most powerful anti-nutrients around. Cereals have developed these toxins to dissuade grain eaters from eating them. Curiously, many seed eaters (which are mainly birds) have developed resistance to lectins. Primates, man included, have never been grain eaters and have no resistance to lectins.

What do lectins do? They are agglomerative molecules that pass into the bloodstream and disrupt the work of any body cell that they attach themselves to. They are powerful provokers of all auto-immune diseases including allergies, asthma, lupus and arthritis. They are even suspected of causing autism in susceptible children.

Worse, lectins, like the Trojan horse, open the back door to the citadel. They cause the gut to be more porous, thus allowing bacteria, funguses and food particles to flood in and create their own mischief.

Ruthlessly cut grains out of your diet if you have a disabling auto-immune disease. Allow about two months for this 'detoxification' regime to work.

There are of course many non-dietary triggers. One of the commonest is stress. Sufferers appear to be allergic to their own stress hormones! Stress reduction technique should be part of any program to alleviate allergic disorders.

But allergens are only one side of the story. The other side is the abnormal reaction of the body. Why does it do that? Some people are less able to deal with some of the 'novelty foods' in the Western diet. Modern inventions like Omega 6 oils, transfatty acids, and other *bad* fats cause the body to make histamines and leukotrienes for example. These are substances that instruct cells to inflame, swell and secrete mucus.

The immune system is depressed by the *bad* fats and oils. It is also undermined by bad food combining. The gut secretes into the blood stream all kinds of harmful bacteria, toxins, funguses and food particles. The immune system goes crazy chasing them down and sweeping them up. Unnecessary tasks. Much better to avoid that and let the immune system get on with the really important job of vacuuming up disease viruses, bacteria and cancer cells.

———— ◆ ————

Don't divert the immune system from its most important job: hunting down viruses, bacteria and cancer cells.

———— ◆ ————

For Food/Immune summary see p. 158.

Diabetes

Adult Onset Diabetes (Type II)

This is a scourge of the Western diet, and it is increasing exponentially. Fully one half of all amputations of hands and feet in the United States are due to diabetes. Similarly, it is a leading cause of blindness. People who are diabetic are much more likely to be obese and have heart disease, kidney disease, high blood pressure, thromboses and strokes.

Why is diabetes increasing so much? Why do Eskimos, Aborigines, Polynesians and American Indians have such fantastically high rates of diabetes as soon as they adopt a Western diet?

What is it about the Western diet that is so harmful? To answer these questions we have to remember that diabetes is due to a dysfunctioning blood sugar control system. Why does it suddenly cease to function properly? Because it has caved in to the onslaught of bloodsugar-making foods. As explained earlier, these are primarily the *bad* carbohydrates that are aided and abetted by the *borderline* carbohydrates.

Secondary causes are dietary errors like the over-consumption of meat, which drives up the demands on insulin secretion and Omega 6 oils which increase insulin resistance of the fat cells.

Diabetes (Type I)

This is a much rarer disease. It is an auto-immune disease. The immune system turns against the insulin-producing cells and destroys their ability to manufacture insulin. Nevertheless, for these sufferers too, diet is a prime means of controlling the progress of the disease. It is just as important to reduce the needs for insulin injections as for Type II diabetes.

Insulin

Cannot diabetes be cured by insulin injections? For many decades it was thought that insulin was a miracle cure. Overnight, a dying person could be 'cured' and given many years of more useful life. This is true.

It has slowly seeped into the consciousness of the medical establishment that there is a big downside. This is the side-effect of insulin, as a hormone, acting on all sorts of other body functions. These give rise to the much higher risk of cardiovascular and myriad other diseases described in Chapter Five.

One big problem with insulin injections is that they present a sudden surge of concentrated hormone to the body. This is nothing like the closely matched secretion, minute by minute, of the pancreas itself.

Perhaps half the number of diabetics do not need insulin injections at all. In spite of that, their risks are hardly lower. They still have insulin levels wildly out of control, and the same risks of disease.

What can be done about this? Very simple, don't put the body under blood sugar stress in the first place. The most important thing a diabetic and pre-diabetic can do is to stop presenting unreasonable demands for insulin. Avoid demanding the body to treat foodstuffs that it was never designed to process. That way insulin levels are kept low all the time.

This is how our ancestors operated, and when Aborigines, Polynesians etc, return to their ancestral eating patterns, their diabetic symptoms improve dramatically. One last comment: exercise has been found to have a marked restorative effect on glucose tolerance. Read Chapter Eleven and make sure that you exercise at least to the minimum shown there.

Be under no illusion, if you are diagnosed with diabetes the battle is to the death. Take no prisoners, make no compromises! There is no time to lose. Go cold turkey on the ideal eating pattern to control diabetes – Natural Eating.

For Food/Diabetes summary see p. 159.

Overweight, Obesity

Everything we know about our prehistoric ancestors is that they were lean. Everything we know about our biology today is that to be overweight is unhealthy.

For our ancestors, food bonanzas were rare. Most of the time they were slightly hungry. We can imagine why. Getting food required work. They did the minimum work necessary for survival. If they finished lunch hungry, they had a choice. Go off for an hour or two and find more food or have a siesta during the heat of the day. There was thus an automatic mechanism controlling the intake of food. You had to really want the food to go to the effort of getting it.

Humans, unlike some creatures, were not living surrounded by their food. We do not have a well-developed satiety reflex. That is to say, our bodies do not have strong signals telling us to stop eating. That never had to be programmed in to us in our Pleistocene past. On the contrary, we have a reflex that tells us to keep eating for as long as there is food around.

───────── ◆ ─────────

The human reflex is to keep eating food while the opportunity is there.

───────── ◆ ─────────

Today of course, in the affluent countries, we are surrounded by food. We can, with no effort, satisfy our desire for food. Today, we need to exercise self-discipline. Fortunately, that self discipline can be exercised not so much on the amount we eat but on what we eat.

How much weight is excess? There is a rule of thumb known as the Body Mass Index (BMI). It is calculated as your weight (in kg) divided by your height (in metres) squared. The same figures applies to both men and women.

Really lean hunter/gatherer societies like the Australian Aborigines or the Bushmen of the Kalahari have BMIs in the range 13 to 19. These peoples have low blood pressure, no heart disease or diabetes, and no cancer.

This seemingly is the ideal. An ideal that is hopelessly out of reach of the average Westerner. Fortunately it is not necessary to reach these very low figures for BMI. The studies show, and modern medical wisdom has accepted, that BMI's in the range 20 to 25 are fine for optimum health. BMI's of 25 to 30 are 'overweight', and already adverse health consequences are setting in. 30 to 35 is 'obese', Over 35 is 'grossly obese'. With increasing levels of obesity, so the health consequences are the more grave.

This table gives some typical values of BMI. The full range is given in the Natural Eating Manual.

What can be done about being overweight? Live like an Australian Aborigine! All right, in the real world that is not possible, so what are the strategies that we can employ?

'Fat makes you fat'. That is true, but that is not the whole story. If it were, Americans, who are paranoid about fat, would be the slimmest people on earth. Instead, in spite of the 20 year drive against fat in the diet, Americans are fatter than ever!

Body Mass Index and Weight			
	Healthy	Overweight	Obese
BMI	20 to 25	25 to 30	30 to 35
Height	**wt. - lb.**	**wt. - lb.**	**wt. - lb.**
5'-3"	113 to 141	142 to 169	170 to 197
5'-8"	131 to 164	165 to 197	198 to 230
6'-0"	147 to 184	185 to 221	222 to 258

No, there is a second factor, *bad* carbohydrates. Having got this far in the book, you will be well aware that the sugars, pastries, breakfast cereals, breads, pastas and potatoes are the new villains of the piece. Indeed as fast as manufacturers have taken fats out of their products, so they have added sugars and other *bad* carbohydrates. The manufacturers are driven by sales, and what the public will buy is foodstuffs that are tasty. And sugars are cheap and easy taste enhancers.

————— ◆ —————

Manufacturers find that sugars are cheap and easy taste enhancers.

————— ◆ —————

It is up to you, the public, to be more discerning. This book will have given you the tools to be so. Read the small print on all the food labels. Ruthlessly exclude fats and bad carbohydrates.

Finally, there are the bad food combinations, especially starch/fat and starch/protein. Why are they so bad? Remember how starch increases the level of insulin in the blood, and how insulin is the fat storage hormone? Eat fat at the same time as starch and insulin will obligingly put the fat on the fast track into your fat cells. Bread and butter, french fries and potato chips are very fattening combinations.

What about the protein? Here there is a double whammy. First, the protein magnifies the starch's effect on insulin production so more of this pesky hormone is there to do its storing work. Second, there is always fat associated with protein. No meat, no fish, no cheese, no egg, is without an accompanying cargo of fat. Even most vegetable proteins (nuts, peanut, soy-bean, garbanzo) are not exempt. So, dishes that mix both protein and starch are very fattening combinations. Examples are: hamburgers (bread and beef), pizzas (pastry and cheese), steak and fries (potato and beef), Spanish omelette (potato and egg).

What if you separate them out? It is better to eat the cheese first then the baguette two hours later than to eat two cheese subs at two hours interval.

In both options, the same amount of food is eaten. In the first case, your insulin levels will have stayed low. There is nothing therefore to encourage the fat in the cheese to be stored in your fat cells. With a bit of luck the fat will be excreted unabsorbed.

But in the second case (the conventional one) the starch in the cheese sub will be levering the fat in the cheese into the fat cells each time you eat it at two hour intervals.

What about alcohol? Rightly, slimmers should be wary of alcoholic drinks and there are three reasons why:

   * Alcohol interferes with the processes that instruct the fat cells to

release their stores into the blood-stream. This is another example of how what we put into our mouths can disrupt body bio-chemistry.

* Alcohol is empty calories.

* Many alcoholic beverages also contain sugar. The sugar is empty calories too, but worse, sugar is a *bad* carbohydrate. It is the sugars in beverages like beer and liqueurs that cause them to be so fattening. Dry wine drinkers are much less vulnerable.

This table gives values of sugar content and total calories for a selection of alcoholic drinks. For comparison, figures for two carbonated beverages are also shown.

Referring to the table, the "sweet and alcoholic" drinks are much more fattening than the "dry and alcoholic" drinks, and it's not just a question of calories, although that is important. The main culprit is the disruption to blood glucose mechanism caused by the sugar content.

The sugar content of various carbonated beverages is now common knowledge. Even so it is salutary to see how just one drink of cola contains 7 teaspoons of sugar. And of course, if they are mixed with spirits (a gin and tonic, for example) then the fattening effect of both drinks is multiplied.

Beverage	drink size	amount	calories	sugar
Sweet and Alcoholic				
beer	bottle/can	12 oz	146	13g
wine, sweet	glass	3 ½ oz	158	12g
liqueur	jigger	1 ½ oz	186	21g
Dry and Alcoholic				
wine, dry, white	glass	3 ½ oz	70	1g
spirit	jigger	1 ½ oz	97	0g
Sweet, non-Alcoholic				
tonic water	can	12 oz	114	29g
cola	can	12 oz	150	35g

In summary, focus your efforts on eating in accordance with the Natural Eating precepts. Don't worry about how much you are eating. Weight loss will take care of itself.

For Food/Obesity summary see p. 160.

Osteoporosis

The question of osteoporosis is one of the most misunderstood in popular nutrition. The authorities are exhorting us to take ever increasing quantities of calcium supplements, while the incidence of osteoporosis (loss of bone calcium) is also becoming epidemic. What is going wrong?

Basically, the conventional wisdom is focusing on only one side of the equation, the consumption of calcium. The other side of the equation is loss of calcium.

Today, our eating patterns cause us to lose calcium from the body faster than we can put it in. It is as though we are trying to fill the bath tub with a tea cup, with the plug out!

The ongoing 'Nurses Study[3]' has been carried out for over 20 years on some 100,000 nurses. It has come up with some interesting results: menopausal women who drink two or more glasses of milk a day are 40% *more likely* to suffer hip fractures than those who drink no milk. Yes, you read that correctly: drinking all that milk for its calcium had the opposite effect to that intended. It had the effect of de-mineralising their bones.

How can this be? The facile reply is to say, "What are grown women doing drinking milk, a foodstuff intended by nature only for unweaned babies?"

Putting such reflections aside, there is a mechanism well known to science called protein induced calciuria. Indeed, it is a scandal that this phenomenon is not taught as a matter of course in the early grades at school. Put simply, excess protein in the bloodstream causes calcium to be lost in the urine. Americans already eat too much protein and, of course, there is protein in milk.

Excess protein wields a double whammy. Protein metabolism leaves the blood acidified (Chapter Four) so the body restores the blood neutrality by using alkaline calcium salts. Where do they come from? From the bones!

The second part of the double whammy is more subtle. Protein has a strange effect on the kidneys. Kidneys are there to filter waste matter from the blood stream. The membrane which controls this has to be finely tuned. It must only let through the waste products. It should not let through the good substances in the blood.

But, under the effect of excess protein, the kidneys lose this fine tuning. They start to leak calcium. The body finishes up with a negative calcium balance and it has to make up the deficit from the stores in the bones.

This is a classic case of a little knowledge being a dangerous thing. We have been like the Sorcerer's Apprentice, meddling with processes that are not fully understood. How many of us learnt at our mother's knee to drink up our milk "because of the calcium"?

We have fallen into the trap of thinking that because a foodstuff contains calcium, then it is a good thing to consume it. In fact there are a number of other considerations.

First of all, just because you've eaten calcium doesn't mean that your body has absorbed it. A large percentage of the calcium we eat passes straight

3 Feskanich; Milk and Bone fractures (Nurses Health Study); AJPH; 1997; 87; 992-997. See bibliography.

through the body and out the other end. The intestines are very good at just taking what the body thinks it needs at that time and letting the excess pass on. Frequently too, the calcium is not bio-available. It is suspected that much of the calcium in cheese, for example, combines with the cheese fat to form insoluble salts which are simply excreted in the stools.

Secondly, just because calcium has got into the blood stream, doesn't mean that the body uses it to build bones. On the contrary, the body is quite capable of laying calcium down just where you don't want it. For example in the arteries, in the heart valves, as nodules in fatty tissue and as painful spurs in the joints.

What is going on? Clinical and epidemiological studies have shown that populations in Asia and in Africa who, although consuming low levels of calcium, nevertheless have a low incidence of hip fracture. This counter-intuitive result indicates that there is some other, powerful factor at work.

This is the key to the osteoporosis question. Some of the most powerful factors in body metabolism are hormones. We know that calcium metabolism is under hormonal control. Our hormonal system, if it is functioning properly, lays calcium down where it is supposed to go. If it is not functioning properly you can have the worst of both worlds, osteoporosis and demineralization of the skeleton at the same time as you are getting atherosclerosis and kidney stones.

But let us look a little closer at what is actually going on in the bones. A bone is made up of living matter in the form of a lattice girder. Its substance is constantly being removed and replaced. In a lifetime its substance will have been turned over several times. There are special cells that build bones, *osteoblasts* and others that dissolve bones, *osteoclasts*.

They are constantly at work, crawling all over the skeleton, removing and replacing bone. It is rather like workmen repainting a girder bridge. As fast as one team strips the old paint off, they are followed by a second team that puts a fresh coat of paint on.

Troubles arise if the stripping team works faster than the painting team, or if the trucker delivering the paint hits a traffic jam, or goes on strike. This is exactly what happens when the bone building team cannot keep up with the bone destroying team. Or when calcium is prevented, by hormones, from being collected from the stores, or from being delivered to where it is needed. This is the most important mechanism to understand about bone health.

There is another important phenomenon. Young people build up bone mass until the age of about 35. Building up and managing of this calcium 'capital' is just as important as managing a retirement account. If you are fortunate enough to be under the age of 35, you have a wonderful chance to build up your maximum bone density. Remember, the deciding factor is hormonal balance, not calcium intake.

Recent studies[4] have concluded that high intakes of micro-nutrients such as potassium, magnesium, vitamin C, fibre and zinc are associated with a higher bone mass. Where are these nutrients found all together and in the right proportions, in fruits! The study concludes that the best strategy for laying down calcium and ensuring good bone health is to eat fruits in abundance.

After the age of 35 your bone capital is vulnerable to depletion. You can choose to run down your bone capital fast, slowly or not at all. Most Americans run their capital down fast. Result: osteoporosis, collapsed vertebrae and hip and femur fractures in old age.

How do we avoid running down this capital? Innumerable studies show that however much you supplement with calcium, there is no improvement in bone density. Indeed, with the bone stripping team outpacing the bone building team due to dietary errors, supplementation does not even slow the rate of bone loss.

On the contrary, over-supplementing on calcium can deplete other minerals in the body such as iron and zinc. It is the Sorcerer's Apprentice syndrome again, meddling in processes that are only half understood and making them worse.

On the other hand, every time you eat some concentrated protein, such as a steak or hamburger, you are presenting a check to the calcium bank which it will pay out of your calcium capital!

The strategy has to be this: stop doing things that run down the capital. What are the most useful things?

1. Eliminate protein excess

The first measure, quite simply, is to not eat an excess of protein. Most Americans overdose on protein. Don't forget it is in nearly everything you eat, including salads and vegetation.

——————— ◆ ———————

Avoid overeating proteins.

——————— ◆ ———————

2. Limit salt consumption

Excess salt causes the kidneys to raid the calcium bank to show this unwanted mineral the back door. Be frugal with the consumption of salt. Eat plenty of fruits. The potassium found in copious quantities both in fruits and vegetables mitigates the effect of excess salt and reinforces calcium metabolism.

4 New et al; Fruit Best for Bone Health; AJCN; 1997; 65; 1831-9. See bibliography.

--------- ◆ ---------
Salt drains calcium from the body.
--------- ◆ ---------

3. Maintain good acid/alkali balance

Consume plenty of plant food. Check back to Chapter Five. Plant foods ensure a good acid/alkali balance, a good hormonal balance and good bone health.

--------- ◆ ---------
A relentlessly acid diet drains calcium reserves
--------- ◆ ---------

4. Consume plenty of micro-nutrients

Studies show that bone-building is dependant on high current intakes of fruits. There are over 20,000 active compounds in fruits and they are far from all being identified and evaluated. Certainly adequate intakes of potassium, zinc, magnesium, fibre and vitamin C are important but not sufficient. You still have to consume the fruits and vegetables themselves to get the benefit of the other bone-building compounds!

Similar studies also show that those who eat a high fruits diet during the first part of life (up to about age 35) accumulate the highest bone mass.

--------- ◆ ---------
Those who eat a high fruits diet have the highest bone mass.
--------- ◆ ---------

5. Avoid overdosing on supplements

Remember the 'law of unintended consequences' in Chapter Four? Vitamin D is an important compound that helps calcium absorption. Mistakenly some people self-medicate and over-do it. Vitamin D over-doses accelerate osteoporosis. As ever, don't try to micro-manage these processes.

--------- ◆ ---------
Go easy on dietary supplements.
--------- ◆ ---------

6. Keep bone-building hormones balanced

Remember that osteoporosis is a disease of hormone imbalances in which the bone destroying cells (osteoclasts) are more active than the bone building cells (osteoblasts). Their respective activities are controlled by hormones. The details are fiendishly complicated and have not been full worked out. Nevertheless, implicated is parathyroid hormone. Too much of it draws calcium out of the bones.

Phosphorous is one compound that excites unfavorable parathyroid activity. It is very prevalent in the Western diet in meat and in colas. People who eat a lot of animal products and/or drink more than the occasional can of cola are undermining their bone health.

———— ◆ ————

Avoid gratuitous phosphorous.

———— ◆ ————

7. Estrogen therapy

If anyone still needed convincing that osteoporosis is a hormonal problem, just consider this: the only medication (as opposed to lifestyle pattern) that is helpful is a hormone, estrogen. Estrogen is used successfully to slow the deterioration in bone health of menopausal women. But why bother? Get your eating patterns right and osteoporosis will be a non-issue. (See also Menopausal women in Chapter Six.)

Some reassuring tips from recent clinical trials:

* Moderate consumption of caffeine, like two cups of American coffee per day, is harmless to calcium metabolism.

* Moderate consumption of alcohol, like one glass of wine per day, can be modestly helpful.

* Modest consumption of fluoride, like the dose from using (but not swallowing) fluorided toothpaste, is helpful to calcium metabolism.

Our hominid ancestors never suffered from osteoporosis and bone demineralisation. The first signs of these diseases only begin to appear in the archaeological record after the sea-change in eating patterns brought about by the farming revolution some 10,000 years ago. Our philosophy is to learn the lessons of evolutionary history and adapt these lessons to the modern world.

For Food/Osteoporosis summary see p. 161.

Digestive Diseases

Indigestion, Constipation, Colic, Irritable Bowel Syndrome, Gastro-Oesophageal Reflux, Colon Cancer, Diverticulosis, Diverticulitis, Piles.

In Robert McCarrison's account (see Chapter Three) of the Hunzas at the turn of the century, he was amazed to find that this small tribe, despite living in the difficult conditions of the high Himalayas, had the most robust health. In particular they only noticed their abdomens when they were hungry!

McCarrison went on to make his fame as director of the Pasteur Research Institute in India. As a research scientist, he investigated all manner of

---

5 On other rat experiments between a Sikh diet (similar to Hunza) and an English diet, the latter's digestive tracts were in a parlous state This is a short extract from the autopsy on one of the 'English' rats. "The case presents an extraordinary contrast to all other ['Sikh']rat's intestines seen up to date. The lumen of the bowel is very much narrowed; the bowel being in its whole course hardly thicker than a piece of string. ... Intestinal stasis is marked; the lower part of the bowel is

aspects of human nutrition. He was ultimately awarded a knighthood in recognition of the outstanding contribution of his efforts. His dietary trials on groups of rats fed either a Hunza diet, a Bengali diet or a working class English diet ring down to us today. The 'Hunza' rats were remarkably free of disease and docile. The other groups suffered from diseases affecting every organ of the body and, further the 'English' rats were neurotic and ill-tempered[5].

McCarrison's work is cited to show how long the scientific community has known that there is something terribly wrong with the 'civilized' diet. Every study since has refined and reinforced our knowledge. And yet the population as a whole is being led by the nose in the opposite direction.

McCarrison concluded his remarks (in the 1921 Mellon lecture) by saying, "Indeed, their buoyant abdominal health has, since my return to the West, provided a remarkable contrast with the dyspeptic and colonic lamentations of our highly civilized communities."

Nothing has changed in over 75 years! Today, if anything the situation is worse, with sales of indigestion remedies at an all-time high.

McCarrison continued, "I don't suppose that one in every thousand of them [the Hunzas] has ever seen a tinned salmon, a chocolate or a patent infant food, nor that as much sugar is imported into their country in a year as is used in a moderately sized hotel of this city [Pittsburgh] in a single day."

How does this relate to digestive problems then? Well, the digestive system is the starting point for everything. Get that wrong and nothing but problems will ensue.

Indigestion

There are only two reasons for indigestion: bad food combining and irritating foods. In the Western diet, the culprit is almost always bad food combining. The remedy is simple, follow the guidelines in Chapter Five. The benefits can be instantaneous.

Common irritating foods are, chilli peppers, pickles, sauerkraut, mustard, curry.

Constipation, Colon Cancer, Diverticulosis, Diverticulitis, Ulcerative Colitis, Irritable Bowel Syndrome, Piles

If you don't have a bowel movement at least once a day you are constipated. This is a completely self-inflicted condition and the remedies are simple. Eat lots of plant food. Why? Because the bacteria in your colon live on the residue from them. The bodies of bacteria form the bulk of feces.

Don't be side-tracked into eating bran products. Bran is abrasive and not at all what the intestinal tract is designed for. On the contrary, it is designed for the 'soft' fibres like pectin and guar that are found in apples

filled with hard, oval feces ...The stomach is very small ... it is filled with coffee ground-like material.... There were papillomatous outgrowths of the stratified epithelium lining the proximal part of the stomach." McCarrison; A Good Diet and a Bad One; IJMR; 1926; 14; 649-54. See bibliography.

and other fruits. Oat bran is an exception. It contains quite a high proportion of soluble fibres. A bowl of oatmeal or oat bran from time to time is OK.

A cautionary note: most people's digestive tracts have been hardened into working only when it is whipped into action by the harsh, insoluble fibres. Shift the emphasis to the soft fibres over a period of several weeks. Give the intestinal muscles time to respond to the subtler signals. Give them time to find again their natural tone.

Primitive societies consume up to 100g of fibre a day from vegetation and fruits. Their intestines are healthy and they never suffer from intestinal diseases. The average American only consumes 11g of fibre per day. Even the recommended minimum[6] of 30g per day is way below the figure for optimum intestinal health.

Remarkably little is known about what exactly happens in the colon. We do know that the bacteria, both good and bad, get busy feeding on the residues and are, accordingly, creating new compounds that are usually reabsorbed into the bloodstream.

So even the 'indigestible' elements of what we eat end up in our bloodstream. Some of these products like acetate, propionate and butyrate have profound effects on both the lining of the intestine and on body biochemistry (such as production of cholesterol).

Incorrect ratios can lead to the conditions known as colitis and irritable bowel syndrome. These two conditions can also be aggravated or triggered by an allergic response. The commonest allergens? Wheat gluten and lactose (milk). Avoiding these two quite unnatural food elements is both rational and curative.

Similar conditions lead to colon cancer, piles and the diverticular diseases. The lining of the intestine is just not designed to have hard, toxic, bacteria laden feces hanging around. Contrary to earlier wisdom, diverticular disease is best treated by eating plenty of fibre – but 'soft' or soluble fibre, the kind that is found in fruits and vegetables.

The full story is being unravelled. But we don't need to know the detail in order to eat wisely. We know from population studies and anthropological studies, what this book tells you. Eat naturally and all these matters turn out right.

Gastroesophageal Reflux:

This is the distressing condition whereby food in the stomach leaks back past the inlet valve into the esophagus. Stomach acid makes painful burns on the esophagus wall. Perhaps the most important cause is bad food

---

6 Many national committees around the world have adopted the recommendations of WHO Europe's publication: James et al, Healthy Nutrition. Preventing Nutrition related diseases in Europe. Copenhagen, WHO Regional Office for Europe, 1988. In the United States, The American Heart Association is also promoting the minimum consumption of 30g/day.

combining (Chapter Five). It puts an unfailing stress on that inlet valve and the hormonal reflexes that control it.

Drinking alcohol before going to bed is another common trigger to this dysfunction.

For Food/Digestive disease summary see p. 162.

Candidiasis

Candida is a kind of yeast that is present in everyone's intestine. It is a malevolent organism, but under healthy conditions it is kept at bay by the 'friendly' bacteria in the intestine which crowd out harmful organisms and the immune system, which is patrolling the body gobbling up foreign bodies.

Candidiasis is the condition caused when the candida organism grows out of control. It causes discharges from various mucus membranes, particularly the mouth and vagina. It also causes gastrointestinal upsets, constipation, itching rectum, gas, cramps and flu-like symptoms.

Candida growth is encouraged by:

  * the foods it likes, notably the undigested particles of sugars and starches

  * the absence of 'friendly' bacteria in the intestine

  * a weak immune system

  * a porous intestine, that allows the yeast to grow and spread throughout the body

  * high levels of sugar in the blood

Strictly eating naturally would, of itself, be all that is necessary. However, it is important to focus on the measures that help this particular condition:

  * reinforce the immune system (see Immune System segment)

  * starve the candida of nourishment

  * ensure good intestinal health (see Digestive Disease segment)

  * provide nourishment to 'good' bacteria

For Food/Candidiasis summary see p. 155.

Moreover

Complexion, Acne, Pimples

No need to draw up a table. Everything said about a good complexion is true. Eat plenty of fruits and vegetables and avoid fried foods. Draw your inspiration from the Natural Eating principles and you will be sure of banishing acne, pimples and a pasty, unhealthy complexion to a distant unpleasant memory.

Cellulite

Dealing with cellulite is a multi-million dollar industry, with all kinds of remedies and fixes being peddled. It is also a problem suffered more by women than men. This is not the place to make extravagant promises about how Natural Eating will cure cellulite. Nevertheless, cellulite is not a characteristic of naturally adapted human beings. Get your body chemistry functioning properly, get your weight down to the ideal and exercise regularly.

Adopt Natural Eating principles and practice the exercise precepts in Chapter Eleven.

Sex, Libido And Fertility

Studies show that a high fat diet diminishes libido and fertility. A diet high in fruits and vegetables is the most helpful. Yes, we do need to eat like rabbits to have the performance of a rabbit.

It is not surprising that our very existence as a species is dependant on a lifestyle identical to that for which we are naturally adapted. Eat naturally and get a new lease on life!

Macular Degeneration

Retinal macular degeneration (a progressive and irreversible deterioration of the retina) is the most common cause of blindness in people over 65. Macular degeneration affects the macula, the part of the eye that distinguishes detail in the centre of the field of vision. Over time, the macula breaks down, causing vision loss. Among other things, the macula is composed of lutein and zeaxanthin.

Studies show that people who consume a high plant diet, notably spinach, cabbage and broccoli, have a 60% lower risk of developing the disease. These vegetables are rich in the two carotenoid anti-oxidant compounds: lutein and zeaxanthin. These compounds filter into the retina and mop up free radicals.

In a more recent study[7], Heidelberg researchers have shown that other foods that contain these compounds are also effective: kiwi, orange peppers, red grapes, zucchini, eggs, even wine. The researchers say that virtually all vegetables have lutein and zeaxanthin.

The Final Word

This chapter goes to great lengths to explain how foods can be helpful or harmful to almost all aspects of our well being. Remember, our feeding patterns are not the whole story. Not every condition is the result of poor

7 Sommerburg et al, Corn, orange, peppers, help preserve vision; British Journal of Ophthalmology 1998;83:907-910.

eating patterns. Not every condition can be cured by the adoption of a healthy eating pattern. Nevertheless, these guidelines will ensure that you have played your cards as well as possible.

Think about this, all the above guidelines are the distilled wisdom of the latest scientific research. It all points in the same direction, to a pattern of eating which is identical to the Natural Eating principles.

It is not surprising that the painstaking unravelling of the workings of the human body is gradually revealing the patterns of eating for which the human race is genetically programmed.

Fridge Door Summary

Candidiasis

Helpful Food Practices

High Vegetation Diet: consume 3 lb. per day of all unrestricted salads and vegetables, (see Table 1, Appendix 1.)
High fruit diet: consume 2 lb. per day of all unrestricted fruits,
(see Table 1, Appendix 1.)

Harmful Food Practices

Bad Food Combining: adopt punctiliously the food-combining rules in Chapter Five.
High Carbohydrate Diet: cut out bad carbohydrates: most cereals, bread, pastries, sugars, honey etc. see Table 3, Appendix 1, and borderline carbohydrates: remaining cereals, dried fruits, banana, rice, etc. (see Table 4, Appendix 1)
Bad Fat Consumption: cut out lard, dripping, butter, cream, butter, milk, palm oil, coconut oil, saturated fat, trans-fatty acid, hydrogenated fat, spreads etc.
Omega 6 Vegetable oil Consumption: cut out sunflower oil, safflower oil, corn oil, peanut oil etc.
High Meat Diet: cut down beef, veal, pork, lamb, chicken, turkey, meat products

Other Harmful Lifestyle Activities

Lack of sleep: depresses the immune system
Lack of exercise: encourages constipation
Alcohol: depresses the immune system
Stress: depresses the immune system

Fridge Door Summary

Rheumatoid Arthritis, Osteo-Arthritis, Multiple Sclerosis, Lupus

Helpful Foods

Omega 3 Oils (moderation): *canola oil, walnut oil, flaxseed oil*
Fatty Fish (moderation): *salmon, tuna, sardine, mackerel*
Fruits and Vegetables: *eat copiously all unrestricted foods, Table 1, Appendix 1*

Harmful Foods

Corn: *sweetcorn, popcorn, hominy*
Wheat: *bread, cornflakes, breakfast cereals generally, cakes, cookies*
Other Grains: *rice, rye, barley, oats*
Milk: *all kinds including buttermilk, skimmed, sour cream, yoghurt*
Omega 6 Vegetable Oils: *corn, safflower, sunflower, peanut, evening primrose and all other oils except those favourable ones mentioned above*
Bad Fats: *lard, dripping, shortening, butter, margarine, trans-fatty acids, hydrogenated fat, palm oil, coconut oil*
Red Meat: *beef (including veal), beef products, lamb, pork, and pork products (bacon, ham, sausage, etc...), cold meats: salami, bologna, etc.*

Suspect Foods
These are common arthritis allergens - try avoiding

Cheese
Other Cereals: *oats, rice, barley, rye*
Eggs
Coffee
Citrus fruits: *orange, grapefruit, lemon, lime*
Tomato and other Nightshades: *potato, bell peppers, chilli pepper, eggplant*
Nuts: *all, particularly peanut*

Other Harmful Lifestyle Activities

Lifting heavy weights: *It has been shown that the regular lifting of heavy weights (either occupationally or for sport) frequently leads to osteo-arthritis. You must stop before the osteo-arthritis establishes itself.*
Obesity: *Being overweight is a strong predictor of osteo-arthritis in the weight bearing joints. Another good reason to trim down.*

Fridge Door Summary

Cardiovascular Diseases

Helpful Foods

Unrestricted Salads and Vegetables: *see Table 1, Appendix 1*
Unrestricted Fruits: *see Table 1, Appendix 1.*
Omega 3 oils (moderation): *canola oil, walnut oil, flaxseed oil*
Oily Fish (moderation): *salmon, tuna, sardine, mackerel*
Nuts (moderation): *particularly walnuts*
Sundry: *tea, ginger, red wine (moderation), hard drinking water*

Harmful Foods

Meat: *cut down consumption of beef, lamb, pork, bacon, sausage, ham, salami and other cold meats*
Dairy: *cut down milk and its products including skimmed milk, buttermilk, yogurt (fat-free or not)*
Other Animal Proteins: *limit consumption of poultry, cheese*
Bad Fats: *cut out lard, shortening, dripping, butter, margarine, spreads, cream, whole milk, full fat yogurt, palm oil, coconut oil, trans-fatty acids, hydrogenated fats*
Omega 6 Vegetable Oils: *cut out sunflower oil, safflower oil, corn oil, peanut oil, evening primrose oil etc.*
Bad Carbohydrates: *cut out cereals, bread, pastries, sugars, honey etc.(See Table 3 Appendix 1)*
Iron: *cut down red meat and iron supplements*
Salt: *cut right down*

Other Harmful Lifestyle Activities

Stress: *stress causes the production of adrenaline and cortisol. Both these in turn promote the production of insulin. Insulin is the villain at the centre of 'syndrome X'. Managing stress manages heart disease. Cortisol and adrenaline also cause cardiovascular damage directly.*
Smoking: *hardly any need to remind people that smoking, amongst many other nasties, causes blood vessels to constrict and promotes the deposition of arterial plaque.*
Dental Diseases: *gum disease and mouth bacteria that proliferate from poor dental hygiene play havoc elsewhere in the body, slipping into the bloodstream and eventually helping form clots that can bring on heart attacks and strokes.*
Alcohol Abuse: *alcoholism promotes cardiovascular disease.*
Lack of Exercise: *people who exercise have higher levels of blood thinning and artery protecting hormones in their blood. Their arteries are more elastic too. Walking 2 miles a day cuts the risk of dying in half for male retirees.*
Obesity: *obesity is an independent predictor of heart disease. Reducing obesity directly reduces risk of cardio-vascular disease.*
Extreme Fatigue: *people who drive themselves to a state of extreme fatigue produce abnormal quantities of plasminogen activator inhibitor (PAI). This impairs fibrinolysis, the body's ability to break down blood clots.*

Fridge Door Summary

The Immune System
Cancer & Auto-Immune Diseases
(allergies, migraine, asthma etc.)

Helpful Foods

Unrestricted Salads and Vegetables: *especially broccoli sprouts; important: broccoli, tomato, onion, garlic; also good: cabbage, cauliflower, brussels sprouts, collard greens, bok choi. See Table 1, Appendix 1.*
Unrestricted Fruits: *apples, oranges, pears, cherries, strawberries, plums, see Table 1, Appendix 1*
Omega 3 oils (moderation): *canola oil, walnut oil, flaxseed oil*
Oily Fish (moderation): *salmon, tuna, sardine, mackerel*
Nuts (moderation): *almonds, walnuts, brazil, hazel*
Sundry: *tea, ginger, red wine (moderation)*

Harmful Foods

Bad Fat: *cut out lard, dripping, butter, palm oil, coconut oil, cream, milk, margarine, spreads, trans-fatty acid, hydrogenated fat*
Omega 6 Vegetable oil: *sunflower oil, safflower oil, corn oil, peanut oil, evening primrose oil, etc.*
Bad Carbohydrates: *cut out cereals, bread, pastries, sugars, honey etc. (see Table 3, Appendix 1*
Red Meat: *cut out beef, lamb, pork, bacon, sausage, ham, salami, bologna etc.*
Meat: *avoid a high meat diet*

Other Harmful Lifestyle Activities

Bad Food Combining
Stress
Smoking
Alcohol Abuse
Lack of Exercise
Overweight
Lack of Sleep
Diabetes
'Adult Onset' Diabetes (Type II)

Fridge Door Summary

Diabetes

Helpful Foods

Salads and Vegetables: *eat copiously all unrestricted salads and vegetables, (see Table 1, Appendix 1)*
Fruits: *eat copiously all unrestricted fruits, apples, oranges, pears, cherries, strawberries, plums, peaches, (see Table 1, Appendix 1).*
Omega 3 Oils: *consume, in moderation, canola oil, walnut oil, flaxseed oil*
Oily Fish: *consume, in moderation, salmon, tuna, sardine, mackerel*
Raw Unsalted Nuts: *consume, in moderation, almonds, walnuts, brazil, hazel*
Legumes: *lentils, beans, garbanzo (chickpea)*

Harmful Foods

Bad Carbohydrates: *cut out most cereals, bread, pastries, sugars, honey etc. (see Table 3, Appendix 1)*
Borderline Carbohydrates: *cut out remaining cereals, dried fruits, etc. (see Table 4, Appendix 1)*
Bad Fats: *lard, dripping, butter, cream, butter, margarine, spreads, milk, palm oil, coconut oil, saturated fat, trans-fatty acid, hydrogenated fat*
Omega 6 Vegetable oils: *cut out sunflower, safflower, corn oil, peanut oil, evening primrose oil*
Animal Flesh: *cut right down*

Other Harmful Lifestyle Activities

Lack of Exercise: *good exercise dramatically improves glucose tolerance*
Overweight: *being overweight is one of the leading indicators of diabetes. Reducing weight is essential.*
Smoking: *diabetics are particularly vulnerable to poor circulation. Smoking causes blood vessels to constrict and reduce even further the circulation to the extremities, feet, fingers, eyes etc.*
Stress

Fridge Door Summary

Overweight and Obesity

Helpful Foods

Salads and Vegetables: eat copiously all unrestricted salads and vegetables, see Table 1, Appendix 1
Fruits: eat copiously all unrestricted fruits: apples, oranges, pears, cherries, strawberries, plums etc. see Table 1, Appendix 1

Harmful Foods

Bad Carbohydrates: cut out most cereals, bread, pastries, sugars, honey, etc. see Table 3, Appendix 1
Borderline Carbohydrates: cut out remaining cereals, dried fruits, banana, rice, etc. see Table 4, Appendix 1
Bad Fats: cut out lard, dripping, shortening, butter, cream, milk, milk products, saturated fat, trans-fatty acid, hydrogenated fat, spreads
Omega 6 Vegetable oils: cut out sunflower, safflower, corn oil, peanut oil etc.
Animal Flesh: cut down beef, pork, lamb, meat products

Other Harmful Lifestyle Activities

Bad Food Combinations: starch/fat and starch/protein combinations are very fattening.
Lack of Exercise: good exercise helps restore malfunctioning glucose and fat metabolism. It's not just the calorie burning that is important.
Alcohol: some people reduce weight even though consuming alcohol moderately, for example a glass of dry wine a day. However, alcohol is empty calories and it inhibits the release of body fat into the bloodstream.
Stress: stress causes the production of adrenaline and cortisol. Both these in turn provoke insulin production - and insulin is the fat storing hormone.

Fridge Door Summary

Osteoporosis

Helpful Foods (as much as you can):

All Unrestricted Salads and Vegetables: especially broccoli, collard greens and bok choi, (see Table 1, Appendix 1)
All Unrestricted Fruits: see Table 1, Appendix 1
Nuts (in moderation): almonds, walnut etc.
Sundry: Fluoride, as obtained for example through using fluorided toothpaste. (Fluoride is toxic in larger doses)

Harmful Foods

Proteins: particularly animal origin
Acid forming starches: see Chapter Five
Sundry: colas, salt

Other Harmful Lifestyle Activities

Lack of Exercise: see Chapter Eleven. Exercise is good; it activates bone building cells.
Alcohol Abuse: Studies show that alcoholics have bone disease. Alcohol directly prevents bone building. Bone so lost is almost impossible to replace.

Fridge Door Summary

Digestive Disorders

Helpful Food Practices

Practice Good Food Combining (Chapter Five)
High Vegetation Diet: *consume 3 lb. per day of all unrestricted salads and vegetables, (see Table 1, Appendix 1)*
High Fruit Diet: *consume 2 lbs. per day of all unrestricted fruits, (see Table 1, Appendix 1)*

Harmful Food Practices

Bad Food Combining: *follow religiously the food-combining rules in Chapter Five*
High Carbohydrate Diet: *cut out bad carbohydrates: most cereals, bread, pastries, sugars, honey etc. (see Table 3, Appendix 1)*
Consumption of Potential Allergens: *cut out dairy products, wheat products etc.*
High Meat Diet: *cut right down consumption of beef, veal, pork, lamb, chicken, turkey, meat products etc.*

Other Harmful Lifestyle Activities

Stress: *stress causes the stomach lining to inflame and function abnormally*
Lack of Exercise: *encourages constipation*
Alcohol Abuse: *encourages constipation and disturbs proper functioning of gastric reflexes*

C h a p t e r   N i n e

Strategies for Implementation

General Principles

Our Pleistocene ancestors were not following any feeding strategies. They just followed what was there and followed their instincts. Their eating patterns would have changed from day to day according to the hazards of foraging. From season to season they would have changed according to the availability of flora and fauna in the environment. Even so, the possible variations would have fallen within quite close limits.

Today, 'what is there' is mostly artificial, and our instincts are readily betrayed by the divorce of taste from nutritional quality. The artful food manufacturers are masters at giving us taste without food value at all. The fluctuations of 'what is there' falls within much, much, wider limits. There is virtually no external discipline of what and how much we eat. So we have to have strategies!

In this chapter we look at typical models for realizing the Natural Eating Pattern. The objective is to give an example of the thought processes, the questioning and the discipline that it is necessary to adopt. Do not get fixated on the patterns described here. Within the boundaries of the Natural Eating precepts there is an infinity of permutations by which you can organize your eating day. Use the examples given here to limber up the brain and get your thought processes working in a new paradigm.

Morning Time

You are being asked to eat a lot of fruit.

You are being asked to eat fruit on an empty stomach.

You are being asked to eat little but often.

A good time to eat fruit is a little while after waking up in the morning. Your stomach is empty (or should be unless you have eaten a really badly combined meal). You can then eat portions of fruit all through the morning until lunch time.

Suppress any prejudices you may have about the desirability of eating a heavy breakfast. It is not desirable! Your body has just awakened from an exhausting night of internal house cleaning. In the morning it is in a mode for eliminating wastes from that process. It welcomes a gradual introduction to the new day with some light tasks such as digesting fruits. Our Pleistocene ancestors knew about that; they didn't start feeding until mid-morning. Don't worry about hunger cravings – there won't be any unless you are a chronic hyperinsulinemic.

You will get to feel a little empty as the morning progresses, so you will then eat another portion of fruit. You eat until the feeling of emptiness is gone. You may have eaten a little or a lot. It doesn't matter nobody is counting. Listen to your body. Don't eat just because it is time to eat. Eat at the time you feel like it and eat the quantity you feel like. That is the way our Pleistocene ancestors ate. It is the way our bodies are designed, and it is, after all, the way our brains are programmed.

Remember that an important part of feeling sated and satisfied has to do with putting our eating apparatus to work. That is feeling the fruit on the lips and teeth. Tearing a bite out, chomping it, grinding it in our mouths and feeling the sensation against our tongues, gums and mouth linings.

There is an added bonus: mouth hygiene is vastly improved due to an improved saliva composition and the mechanical scouring action of the chewing process.

Mid-morning

You can continue eating your fruits. Or you can shift to something else temporarily. A quick-fix dish of lentil and tomato, or an avocado pear, or a big bowl of vegetable soup. Get used to making extra large quantities of everything so that the fridge/freezer has a ready supply of easily accessed foods.

Now it is Lunch time and Afternoon:

You are being asked to eat lots of vegetables.

You are being asked to eat little starch or protein.

You are being asked not to mix starch and protein.

You are being asked to eat little but often.

A suitable choice might be a mixed salad. An appropriate quantity will be 12 oz. Measure it until you are used to eyeballing the quantities - it's larger than you are used to! Get in the habit of thinking that a salad is often in two parts. There will, on the one hand, be the salad vegetables proper, comprised uniquely of foods from Table 1 - Good Foods to be Eaten in Bulk. On the other hand there will be some additions of either protein or starch.

Tuna, chicken breast, veggie burger or cheese for example can be either added to the salad or eaten as a side dish. The same goes for the possible addition of sweetcorn or pasta.

Take care to avoid the bad combination of both protein and starch. A protein dominated dish like salad Niçoise[1] for example is best without the potato. You are eating 12 oz. of salad, plus about 3 oz. of proteins. (Remember that Acid/Alkali Balance in Chapter Five?) Often potato is added to the recipe. You are in charge of the meal, so get into good habits. Leave the potato out.

Again get used to the quantities of the protein or starch. This time they are smaller than you think. (See Table 2: Good Foods to be Eaten in Controlled Quantities in Appendix 1.)

Use the standard homemade salad dressing, consisting of canola oil plus a dash of lemon juice or vinegar and a pinch of salt and pepper. If you have time, a clove of crushed garlic is good. (See Sample Recipes, Chapter Twelve)

Preferably, eat the salad before the side dish. This fast-tracks the vegetables through the gateway of the antrum. That way your appetite will be more readily satisfied on the healthiest part of the meal. Eating the low density plant food takes time. This allows the satiety reflex time to catch up and make you feel replete. The sides can then take their time in the stomach's acid bath.

Through the afternoon, you may begin to feel hungry. For example, you will have, ready prepared in your fridge, some raw broccoli, cauliflower and baby carrots. You will also have some pots of preservative-free dips such as guacamole and salsa. That's it - a raw vegetable dip.

This is only one solution. More conventionally, fill some pockets of whole-wheat Pita bread with the remains of the salad or other fillings such as ratatouille or alfalfa sprouts. This makes a wholesome and enjoyable sandwich.

Note the strategy, a Pita pocket, unlike a conventional sandwich, is capable of holding more than three times its own weight in plant filling. This keeps the ratio of plant food to starch in the healthful proportion.

Both these kinds of snack are easily transportable if you are out and about. Get used to taking your fuel with you when you are away from home for several hours. Above all, overcome any inhibitions you may have about pulling it out and eating it when the occasion calls.

———— ◆ ————

Get used to taking your fuel with you when away from home.

———— ◆ ————

1 Salade Niçoise of France combines lettuce with green beans, olives, tuna, potato, tomatoes, and anchovies, all dressed with olive oil and vinegar.

Come Dinner Time, Then What?

It's the same decision-making process as at lunchtime. This time you decide to do some cooking. Maybe 1 lb. of stir-fried vegetables accompanied by a two egg (2 oz) omelette. Or a vegetarian burger (go for one which is constituted mainly from vegetable). It's as easy as that. The stir-fry can be ready frozen, but throw away any accompanying sauce and season with garlic and soy sauce. Note that we are escaping the tyranny of the starter, main course, dessert, regimen. Just the one course. As ever, try to eat the vegetables before anything else.

If you fancy it, a glass of dry, red wine is OK.

Now it's close to bed-time and you feel like some supper.

Believe it or not, there is quite a choice. If there is a sufficient gap after the last meal (see the Golden Rules). It could be a fruit (as much as you like). If not, it could be 2 oz of nuts, almonds are good, or even the remains of the stir-fry. Avoid bad carbohydrates this late in the day. The hormonal reaction is inimical to a good night's sleep, but worse, it interferes with the body's nighttime repair processes.

Bad carbohydrates before bedtime interfere with nighttime cell renewal, you wake up tired to boot.

If you fancy it, have a mug of cocoa (100% cocoa powder) made with water and sweetened with aspartame. (See the recipe in Chapter Twelve.) Definitely avoid any "hot chocolate" drinks. You only have to read the fine print to see how little cocoa and how much junk and filler is in them.

It is even possible to have 1 oz of that dark, bitter European chocolate. It should have the highest percentage of cocoa possible. Read the fine print. If cocoa comes before sugar on the list, then this is already acceptable. Really good varieties will give the percentage of cocoa indicated. e.g. cocoa solids 65%.

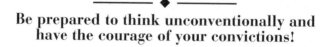

Be prepared to think unconventionally and have the courage of your convictions!

Eating Away From Home

It is one thing to get organized at home for eating naturally but it is quite another matter when away from home. However, by planning ahead, being assertive and being prepared, it is quite possible to stay close to the ideal regimen.

Restaurants

In reasonable quality restaurants, it is relatively simple to find items on the menu which can form the basis of a meal, because there will still be clarifications and negotiations to be conducted with the waiter. Decide first whether you are going to make it a protein meal or starch meal.

Then you start the questions. "What exactly does the salad have in it? I don't want any croutons, pasta, rice, fruit..." or, "I don't want any cheese, nuts, fruit." Then you ask,

"What is the salad dressing?"

Waiter	"Ranch"
You:	"What is in it?"
Waiter:	"I don't know, it comes out of a big jar."
You:	"In that case I would like the oil and vinegar cruet, thank you very much."

So it goes on, until you have selected the starter, main course and dessert.

You will have paid close attention to the vegetables that accompany the main course. You will refuse potatoes, French fries and rice which are often offered as "vegetables." You will ascertain that green beans, or broccoli, or spinach or any other green vegetable is available and you will ask for *double* portions.

If it is a *protein* meal, you will not eat any of the bread from the bread basket. You will leave at the side of the plate any sweet corn that may have intruded in spite of the negotiations.

If it is a *starch* meal, and if you are feeling in a crusading mood, try asking for whole-wheat pasta, or whole-grain rice. Restaurants are usually puzzled by this request, but if enough people ask for it they might change their ways. This is one more area where the tide of inappropriate feeding habits can be rolled back.

Spaghetti sauces are problematic. No meat sauces of course, that would be a bad starch/protein combination. A tomato sauce is fine but some people are troubled by its acidity. It can be an awkward combination with starch. Better, the Mediterranean sauces are good, If the restaurant has an olive tapenade sauce (see recipe in Chapter Twelve) for example, that is fine. If not, go for a simple dressing of garlic/olive oil.

The difficulty with a starch-based meal is that the starches are almost always *bad* carbohydrates and there are lots of opportunities to be tempted. There will be the side of garlic bread and the dessert list of cakes, pastries and other assorted hyperinsulinemia shots.

Either way, most of the desserts will be off limits. However, they may have an excellent cheese board. After a protein meal, choose a nick of gourmet cheese and wash it down with a glass of dry red wine. Remember, no bread or biscuits with the cheese!

After either type of meal a low ice-cream or sorbet could be fine. So is chocolate mousse. Ask about the ingredients. There is usually sugar, so eat just a modest amount.

One type of fruit that can safely be eaten by most people after a meal are the red berry fruits, strawberry and raspberry.

When you have finished such a meal you can congratulate yourself. You have eaten healthily and within the margins of tolerance.

Fast Food Outlets

Eating in fast food restaurants is just the same only harder.

Resign yourself to ordering the burger and throwing away the bun. Find a salad if you can. Some keen practitioners carry a bottle of their own salad dressing.

Or, eat the all-day breakfast, eggs, tomatoes, mushrooms. Avoid the sausage, steak, French fries, baked potato, hash-browns, rice, toast, waffles, corn syrup or muffins.

Or, eat a pizza, vegetarian one, and definitely no cheese, eggs or anchovies (avoid starch/protein combinations). Find some salad if you can.

Many fast food restaurants have salad bars. This is good news and with care one can eat reasonably correctly. They do tend to drench the salads in sweetened dressings. Often they mix in fruit, or combine starches and proteins. Be selective. Pick out and put aside the offending ingredients. Be suspicious of the salad dressings. They are invariably made with low quality ingredients, fillers and dosed with sugars. Do the best you can. You are only one meal away from redressing the imbalance!

Dinner Parties

In some ways this is the hardest situation to manage. You don't want to put your hosts under pressure; you want to be invited another day.

If you know your hosts well, it is all right to call in advance and mention that you have special dietary requirements. Say you prefer fish over red meat. (Today this is no longer an exceptional request). Say you don't like to eat fruit after a meal. Say you like green salads. Say you like lots of green vegetables.

Then tuck into your meal and enjoy it for what it is. You will certainly have to compromise, but then your basic eating habits are natural and healthy and the occasional lapse is not going to be the end of the world.

The main priority is to avoid eating in a way that you know, from your own experience, will upset you.

If you don't know your hosts well, or the dinner party is a set menu, then it is best to act defensively. You don't want to go hungry and you don't want to be churlish. So before setting off, eat a light meal of vegetable matter. Salad, vegetable or whatever. Then, when you get to your dinner eat lightly. Enough to preserve appearances and to flatter the cook. The "allergy excuse" is always accepted when you want to leave a significant portion on your plate. People also understand if you are watching your waist-line and don't want to eat much of the dessert. You will find that you escape from this challenge in pretty good order.

How to Get Your Priorities Right

The next chapter is the *'Ten Steps to Success'*. It sets out the actions to concentrate on step by step. Remember that the objective is to get your body operating at optimum health and efficiency. Remember, you don't have to be perfect, just good enough. Once you have reached this stage, it will be able to support more 'lapses'.

This is where you can decide to indulge in some 'minor sins'. For example, you can have a half bottle of wine with your dinner; eat a steak from time to time, or have a piece of key-lime pie on Sundays. On various feast days like Thanksgiving and Christmas you don't have to refuse the pumpkin pie or the plum pudding and custard. After all this is what you have been saving up for. Just don't overdo it!

You can even indulge in the really *bad* carbohydrate from time to time (like waffles and maple syrup, or ice-cream sundae). But do be very careful and disciplined. *Bad* carbohydrate is an addictive drug and it is only too easy to end up at the bottom of the slippery slope.

———— ◆ ————

Bad carbohydrate is an addictive drug. It is too easy to end up at the bottom of the slippery slope!

———— ◆ ————

Do listen to your body. It will surely protest if you overstep its tolerance level. Allergies will reappear, weight will come back on, you will be troubled by digestive troubles. And, of course, you will never know to what extent you are jeopardizing your long term health.

You will be surprised to find that, after a while on this programme, your tastes change. Steaks are unimportant or even repulsive, and you will contemplate a defrosted supermarket chocolate cake with the same enthusiasm as you would a cockroach floating in your soup.

Trust those hard won reflexes! Don't force your way past them and back into the zone of bad habits.

How to Survive in the Real World

The foregoing guidelines are a counsel of perfection. In the real world compromises have to be made.

Have the courage of your convictions in restaurants. Ask exactly what goes into the various dishes. Have them leave out unwanted matter. Cheese for example intrudes into almost everything. Exchange the hash browns for extra green vegetables or a salad.

You really do have to discipline yourself not to be tempted by really bad combinations and junk ingredients such as hamburgers, hot dogs, pizzas and fish 'n' chips.

There will be other 'lapses'- bad combinations, junk food etc. Save them for when you don't want to embarrass the host at a dinner party. Or when you want to have a treat, say, once a week. Monitor how they affect your health and digestion.

Some faulty combinations are 'minor sins', like eggs on toast (protein/starch); macaroni cheese (starch/protein). Just don't overdo it. Monitor what they do to your digestion and *weight*. Apart from potentially causing digestive difficulties, they are fattening combinations.

——————— ◆ ———————

Starch/protein combinations are fattening.

——————— ◆ ———————

The consumption of alcohol is deprecated. In the real world a sugarless alcohol (see table in the Obesity/Overweight section of Chapter 8) such as dry wine, can be drunk in moderation as the meal progresses. Beer, cocktails and liqueurs, being loaded with free sugars, are to be avoided. Dry spirits may be drunk frugally on a full stomach.

Avoid drinking alcohol on an empty stomach. If you are caught unawares with an early cocktail, line your stomach with a protein nibble (cheese cubes, olives). Or, better still, if they have a vegetable dip eat the vegetable, be suspicious of the dip.

C h a p t e r   T e n

Ten Steps to Success

One theme of this book is that every movement in the right direction will bring its benefits. How are you to know which is the right direction? This chapter tells you how.

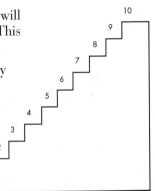

Another theme of this chapter is that most people have a completely erroneous idea of what is important. It is sad to see a health-conscious eater making great efforts to eat in ways that, in reality, are counter-productive. This is an enormous misapplication of that precious resource - willpower.

Our willpower is finite and needs to be delivered where it will do most good. In other words, how are you to prioritize? This chapter tells you how.

◆

This chapter points you in the right direction and prioritizes which steps to take first.

◆

The information is presented sequentially as the steps of the staircase. Each step is in priority order. Step one has the highest priority; step ten the lowest priority.

Put in place the habits in step one and then move on to step two. Thus, step by step you will gradually modify your habits in the right direction. Take it at the pace that is comfortable for you. You can even decide to stop at some intermediate stage.

Each step is a summary of the more detailed advice given in the body of the book. If in doubt refer back to the book.

There follows a series of tables giving examples of foodstuffs in the various categories used in the step descriptions.

One final point before embarking on the staircase:

When you see normal font (like this) that means that the advice is final. It won't be mentioned again, but you are still supposed to practicing that habit right through the following steps.

When you see italic font (like this) that means that the advice is an intermediate measure. A later step will turn the screw tighter.

Examples of Terms used in the Staircase.

Examples of Hard Proteins		
Table 1 **Difficult**	Table 2 **Acceptable**	Table 3 **Good**
bacon	cheese	salmon
beef	chicken breast	tuna
bratwurst	crab	mackerel
chicken	duck breast	sardine
cold meats	eggs	herring
frankfurter	goose, lean	(only)
ham	lobster	
hamburger	mussels	
lamb	oysters	
pork	prawns	
salami	shrimp	
sausage	turkey breast	
turkey	wild game	
veal	other fish	

Examples of Soft Proteins		
Table 4 **Suitable**		Table 4 **Good**
legumes:	*nuts(raw):*	walnut - raw
black bean	almond	(only)
garbanzo[1]	brazil	
haricot bean	cashew	
kidney bean	cob[2]	
lentils	pistachio	
navy bean	pine	
peanut (raw)	other nuts	
peas		
soy bean		
soy protein		

SuperVeg
Table 6 **Excellent**
broccoli
broccoli sprouts
brussels sprouts
cabbage
cauliflower
collard greens
turnip greens

Examples of Fats & oils		
Table 7 **Good**	Table 8 **Acceptable**	Table 9 **Bad**
canola[3] oil - best for everyday use	cocoa butter	butter
flaxseed oil - good condiment	duck fat	coconut cream
hemp oil[4] - good condiment	goose fat	coconut oil
olive oil[5]	soy bean oil	corn oil
spreads - from canola oil[6]		cream
walnut oil - good condiment		hydrogenated oils
		lard
		margarine
		palm oil
		peanut oil
		safflower oil
		shortening
		sunflower oil
		transfatty acids

For Examples of **Bad, Borderline, Good Carbohydrates,** see Tables 5, 6 and 7, Appendix 1.

1 Also known as chick pea.
2 Also known as hazelnut or filbert.
3 Also known as rapeseed oil or colza oil.
4 Hemp oil has an excellent fatty acid profile. This little known oil is becoming more available.
5 Olive oil has no essential fatty acids, but it is health neutral, tasty and heat resistant. Don't let it crowd out the use of the other good oils.
6 Trans-fatty acid free and hydrogenated fat free spreads made uniquely from canola are more easily found in health food stores.

Definition of Terms

'Hard' Proteins are chiefly of animal origin. They require a longer stay in the stomach, especially if they are well cooked. Their cargo of sulfur and other compounds present a challenge to the body's detoxification system.

'Difficult' Proteins are hard proteins that have additional drawbacks, usually a high proportion of bad fats.

'Acceptable' Proteins are 'hard' proteins that are not harmful in modest servings.

'Good' Proteins (hard or soft) have a good essential fatty acid profile. They are important to the body.

'Soft' Proteins are chiefly of vegetable origin. They pass through the stomach faster than hard proteins. Their detoxification is less of a load on the body's biochemistry.

'Suitable' Proteins are 'soft' proteins that are fine for human consumption even if, like the legumes, we are not naturally adapted to them, or like the nuts that have to be eaten in controlled quantities because of their high fat content.

'SuperVeg' are uncommonly helpful to human biochemistry. The various trace compounds have a powerfully helpful effect on many troublesome degenerative diseases.

'Nuts' are nuts from trees. Eat raw and unsalted.

'Good Fats & Oils' have a good essential fatty acid profile. They have little or no injurious fats. It is good to consume a minimum of 5g (1 tsp.) per day. Nevertheless they are still fat and should be consumed in modest quantities. Olive oil's chief merits are that it does no harm and it is heat resistant.

'Acceptable Fats & Oils' have fatty acid profiles that are not injurious to health. They are still fat and should be consumed in modest quantities. Cheese makes this category because its bad fats are less bioavailable.

'Bad Fats & Oils' have a fatty acid profile that is definitely unhelpful to health.

'Bad Carbohydrates' put a big stress on the body's blood-sugar control mechanism.

'Borderline Carbohydrates' put a moderate stress on the body's sugar-control mechanism.

Step 1

Start Here

This step is the most important. Most of the changes are not difficult. Much of it is the simple exchange of one food by an equal substitute. Other changes are to do with the order in which foods are eaten. None of it demands a lot of willpower.

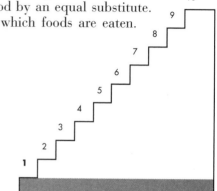

Food Combining:

- Eat fruit on its own.
- Eat melon alone.

Cooking:

- Prefer blanching, stir-frying or steaming.

Fruit:

- *Eat at least 1 apple/day.*

Bad Carbohydrates:

- Replace white bread, rice and pasta - by brown.
- Replace sugar by aspartame.
- Replace regular colas and soft drinks by 'diet' versions.

Bad Oils:

- Replace all other fats and oils by 'Good Fats and Oils (Table 7).

Hard Proteins:

- *Eat no more than 1 serving per day.*

Step 2

Food Combining:

- Eliminate 'hard' protein/starch combinations.

Vegetation:

- Eat at least 1 salad per day.

Dairy:

- *Replace whole milk by skimmed - no more than 1 cup/day.*

Bad Carbohydrates:

- *Pastries no more than 3 servings per week.*
- *Beer - no more than 1 can per day.*
- *French fries - no more than 3 servings per week.*

Hard Proteins:

- *Difficult proteins - no more than 3 servings per week.*
- Good proteins: (oily fish) eat 2 oz. 3 times per week (optional).

Good Proteins generally:

- Eat up to 3 servings per week.

Step 3

Food Combining:
• Eliminate soft protein/starch combinations.

Cooking:
• *Deep fry no more than once per week.*

Bad Carbohydrates:
• *Breakfast cereals - have 3 cereal-free days/week.*

Dairy:
• *Yogurt - only unsweetened, non-fat.*

Acceptable Protein:
• *Eggs - no more than 8 per week.*

Fruit:
• *Eat at least 1 apple + ½ lb. other fruit per day.*

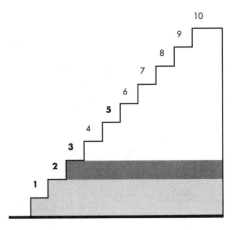

Step 4

How to Eat:
• Keep meals simple.

Vegetation:
• *Eat at least 1 lb./day of salads & vegetable.*

Dairy:
• *Cream - no more than 3 servings per week.*

Bad Carbohydrates:
• Eliminate all processed fruit juices.

Salt:
• Reduce salt added in cooking to bare minimum.

Soft Proteins:
• *Eat at least 3 servings per week.*

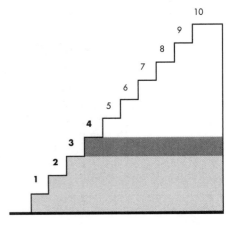

Step 5

How To Eat:
- Eat little but often.

Fruit:
- *Eat at least 2 apples + 1 lb. other fruit per day.*

Dairy:
- *Cheese - no more than 10 oz per week.*

SuperVeg (Table 6 this Chapter):
- *Eat at least 3 servings per week.*

Soft Proteins:
- Tree Nuts - eat at least 2 oz., but no more than 3 oz. per day.

Bad Carbohydrates:
- *Confectionery - no more than 2 times per week.*

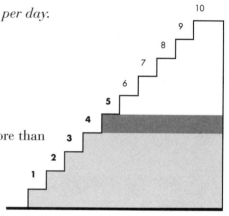

Step 6

Cooking:
- *Deep-fry no more than once per month.*

Vegetation:
- *Eat at least 1½ lb. of salads and vegetables per day.*

Bad Carbohydrates:
- *Beer - no more than 3 cans per week.*
- Potato - eliminate French fries.

Hard Proteins:
- Difficult: no more than one serving per month.
- *Acceptable: no more than 2 servings per week.*

Dairy:
- *Replace the skimmed milk by non-dairy substitutes.*

Step 7

Fruit:
• *Eat at least 2 apples + 1½ lb. other fruit per day.*

Bad Carbohydrates:
• *Bread - eat no more than 2 slices per day.*

Dairy:
• Cream - eat no more than 1 serving per week.

Salt:
• Add strict minimum at the table.

Acceptable Proteins:
• Eggs: no more than 6 per week.

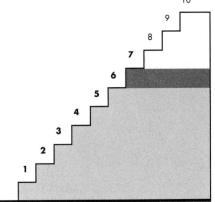

Step 8

Put in place the habits of Step 8 and you have reached the plateau where you can start to relax. This is your body's comfort zone. Steps 9 and 10 are more a question of fine tuning to achieve a level of grand-master!

SuperVeg:
• Eat at least 6 servings per week.

Bad Carbohydrates[7]:
• Low Density – no more than 8 oz. per day.
• Medium Density – no more than 4 oz. per day.
• High Density – no more than 3 oz. per day.

Dairy:
• *Cheese - no more than 3 oz., 3 times per week.*

Soft Protein:
• Eat about 3 oz. per day.

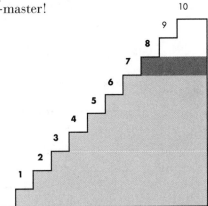

7 Keep these to separate meals and separate from the Borderline Carbohydrates in step 9.

Step 9

Vegetation (vegetables and salads):
• Eat at least 2 lb per day.

Borderline Carbohydrates[8]:
• Low Density – no more than 12 oz once per day.
• Medium Density – no more than 8 oz per day.
• High Density – no more than 4 oz, once per week.

Dairy:
• Strictly limited to the occasional use in cooking.

Artificial Sweeteners:
• Reduce to strict minimum.

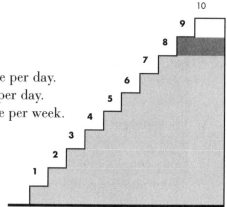

Step 10

Phew! You've made it to the top. Keep this up and you will be sure of making the most of your health potential. Remember, no need to get anxious if occasionally you have to compromise. You are only one meal away from putting it right again. You can anyway circulate within the body's comfort zone represented by Steps 8 to 10.

General:
• Prefer organic foods wherever available.

Bad Fats & Oils:
• Eliminate entirely.

Good Oils:
• No more than 2 tbs per day.

Artificial Sweeteners:
• Eliminate entirely

Dairy:
• Eliminate entirely

8 Keep these to separate meals and separate from the Bad Carbohydrates in step 8.

Chapter Eleven

Exercise

Looking at our genetic programming is a powerful technique for identifying the optimum way to feed ourselves. This same technique can be applied to other aspects of our lifestyles. One of these is exercise. What is our genetic programming for exercise?

The Genetic Foundations

* Over the millions of years of evolution, what were the patterns of physical activity practiced by our species?

* What will that tell us about the amount of exercise we should be getting today?

Surprisingly, we can work out a lot about the physical activity of our Pleistocene ancestors. First of all we know how they must have foraged for food, how far they travelled, how fast, and even their muscular development.

Further, by studying contemporary forager tribes, we can see how they organized themselves on a daily basis.

A typical Pleistocene group consisted of thirty-five to forty-five people, roughly equally divided between men and women. This group would camp in one place for a few days and then move on make another camp 10 to 20 miles away. They carried very little with them, but they still had to walk all the way! They moved, not for the fun of it, but because they had to. The terrain would be open savannah-type grassland in the tropics of East Africa.

While camped, each day the group would split up to forage for food. The women, children and old men went off in one party, foraging for roots, fruits, tubers, berries and easily caught bugs and animals. This party, on average, covered about 5 miles. They leisurely walked and rested from time to time. After about four to five hours they were done. The children walked too and, a lot of the time, scampered about and chased each other as well as the lizards and beetles. Babes in arms, of course, were carried.

It is estimated that the average adult female energy expenditure was 600 kcal per day on physical activity. This compares to 230 kcal for today's sedentary female office worker.

The able-bodied men went off, chiefly looking for small game, but would also be collecting other edible matter on an opportunistic basis. This party would cover more ground during the day – 9 to 12 miles on average. Part of the time they would be running or jogging, to chase and trail potential game. Most of the time, they too would be finished after about four to five hours. However on rarer occasions they might be away for as much as 48 hours tracking a wounded animal.

It is estimated that their daily expenditure of energy was over 1,000 kcal. Compare this to the 306 kcal of the average sedentary male office worker.

There are, therefore, two patterns, one for each gender:

Females would pass their lives exercising to a moderate extent and low intensity.

Males started their lives with the female pattern, graduated to the masculine pattern for most of their lives (vigorous and more sustained physical activity) and then tapered off to feminine levels again in old age.

How does this chime with what we know about human biology today? It fits very well. Evidence is that women do not need to exercise so long or so hard as men to maintain their health. Men need more vigorous physical activity to maintain health. From the world of track athletics we know that men are better built for endurance running.

What happened to our ancestors in old age? What is striking is that old people stayed physically active until their very last days. They were athletes right to the end. The end would come when they could no longer keep up with the group when it moved camp some 10 miles away. The infirm person would be left behind, propped up under a bush, to await the arrival of the jackals and other predators. In this harsh existence, there was no room for people who put the survival of the group at risk.

———— ◆ ————

Just imagine how average life expectancy would drop today, if anyone who couldn't walk 10 miles were left for dead!

———— ◆ ————

So what are we to make of this? Everything we know about peoples or individuals who get this amount of physical activity demonstrates that, as a result, they have better health than they would otherwise have had. Note the qualification 'than they would otherwise have had'. Exercise by itself is not enough. Other lifestyle activities can be even more important in determining good health, notably non-smoking and good eating habits.

The big question is are there any vital body functions that *depend* on physical activity? Yes, indeed there are. Studies, going from those on bed-ridden people to astronauts, all point to a number of conditions brought about by a lack of physical activity. We are not like the bear for example that can stay immobile for 6 months (while hibernating) without suffering health consequences.

What are the consequences for human health then, of physical inactivity? Let's look at some of them.

Exercise and Health Factors

Bone demineralisation and fractures

This condition is multi-faceted, but all the evidence suggests that regular physical activity improves bone structure, its volume and thereby resistance to fracture. Elderly women can benefit from as little as one hour per week of lower-intensity activity - 42% lower risk of hip fracture and 33% lower risk of vertebra fracture[1]. The rhythmic jolting associated with walking/jogging, excites the bone building cells (osteoblasts) into raising their tempo. In young people the bone builders work faster than the bone strippers and bone mass increases. Even in older people the bone builders will work harder and fall less far behind the bone strippers.

Rheumatism, arthritis and joint stiffness

Regular activity of the kind practiced by our Pleistocene ancestors encouraged cartilage maintenance, lubrication and renewal of the wearing surfaces. Dysfunctional joints are due in large part to not giving them enough to do. If you don't use it, you lose it!

Syndrome X

This is the collective name given to a quarto of 'diseases of civilization': high blood pressure, coronary artery disease, obesity and diabetes. They all have a common link – high insulin levels. Yes, our old nemesis of insulin rears its ugly head. Low exercise levels mean that more insulin has to be secreted to handle a given glucose load. Result: more insulin floating around creating mischief. (See Chapter Five.)

Lower leg circulation

There is an artery that passes through the ball of the foot. As you walk or run this artery gets alternately compressed and released. The general effect is that of a pump. Walking/running helps pump blood through the lower leg. Without it the lower leg gets poor circulation and is prone to deep vein thrombosis.

Are you one of those people who, after a little while sitting at a desk or table, find their knees jogging up and down? This too, is a natural reflex

1 Gregg et al; Ann Intern Med 1998;129:81-88,133-134.

helping to maintain lower leg circulation.

Lymphatic circulation

As handmaiden to our blood circulation, we have a secondary system of circulation, known as the lymphatic system. This is responsible, in part, for transporting the products of digestion to other parts of the body; bringing immune system killer cells to parts of the body under attack and flushing away debris and toxic matter. Unlike the blood, which is pumped around the body by the heart, the lymphatic system does not have a pump of its own. It relies on the general flexing of muscles to do the job. Lack of physical activity means sluggish lymphatic circulation and a host of maladies linked to that.

Cosmetic reasons

We are all, every single one of us, descended in an unbroken chain of ancestors who have all successfully found a mate and reared their children. Couples who got together to have children and didn't, failed for a number of reasons. Accidents, sickness, infertility all take their toll. But the bottom line is that they didn't have any offspring.

It follows that we are descended from people who have been successful in having children. They were successful because they were lucky and because they were healthy. Not much can be done about luck, accidents and so on, but over the long term our ancestors will have been slightly better at picking healthy mates. We are *programmed* to recognize a healthy prospective mate. That, to a large extent, is the substance of the 'chemistry' that sparks between two people who are attracted to each other. 'Looking good' is an important part of successful human reproduction.

Even if you are not looking for a mate, 'looking good' gives pleasure to others. Film stars make their fortunes out of people's hunger to cast their eyes on good looking people. The exact nature of the good looks changes with the mood of the times, but the fundamentals do not. No one is going to make it as a heart throb if they are giving off an air of general ill health. Glowing complexion, vibrant muscle tone and an energetic demeanour are attractive in their own right. We are genetically programmed to find them so.

Self preservation

In the world of our ancestors, they did a lot of walking and running because they had to. It was a matter of survival. It was the means by which they got their dinner. If they were unsuccessful in getting dinners they *became* dinner for another creature!

In today's world such automatic sanctions for lack of physical fitness are rare. It is quite possible to live a lifetime as a couch potato and never be embarrassed by a situation where your physical abilities are found wanting. But just think about this: in an air crash, do you want to be the last one to get out of the emergency door?

Longevity

Recent, carefully controlled Finnish studies[2] over many years on identical twins have demonstrated what many people have long suspected, that physically fit people live longer than those who are not.

In this study, it was found that in any given period, 'Sedentary' people were 1.3 times as likely to die as the 'occasional' exercisers and nearly twice as likely to die as the 'conditioning' exercisers. The figures were the same for both men and women.

The exercise criteria were extremely modest.

* 'Conditioning' exercisers exercised for a minimum of 30 minutes, 6 times a month.

* 'Occasionals' exercised even less than the 'conditioners' but did some regular exercise.

* 'Sedentary' people claimed not to exercise at all.

We do not know the effect on longevity if regular physical activity is raised to the level of our prehistoric ancestors, but the suspicion has to be that it is yet further improved.

Stress, depression and mood

Anecdotal evidence is now confirmed by an understanding of human biochemistry. Physical exercise has a beneficial effect on a whole range of hormones that regulate mood.

Exercise modulates hormones that act on serotonin receptors helping to lift depression. It brakes the production of stress hormones such as cortisol and adrenaline. Reducing these two hormones not only reduces feelings of panic and stress, it also reduces the knock-on effect, production of insulin and all the damage that follows.

Finally, carried to an extreme, endurance runners reach a 'high' where their bodies are producing morphine-like substances, giving them a tremendous feeling of well-being.

───── ◆ ─────

Exercise is good to improve feelings of well-being.

───── ◆ ─────

Optimum Exercise Pattern

So just like for eating, it is possible to identify the most favourable pattern

2 Kujala; [Exercise linked to longevity]; JAMA 1998;279:440-444.

of exercise for human beings.

Having read the foregoing you will not be surprised to hear what the ideal level of physical activity is:

* women, children and old men – walk five miles per day, every day.

* able bodied men – walk and run 9 to 12 miles per day every day.

All the studies confirm that these exercise patterns are the optimum for good health. Indeed anyone doing that today is considered to have a high level of fitness. For our ancestors, it was just the norm for everyone.

But what are we to do in the modern world? For most of us it is just not practicable to spend four hours a day exercising. Is it really necessary to exercise so much? Are other forms of exercise more helpful?

The hard answer is that you get out what you put in. The good news is that the response is not linear. At the start you get a lot of benefit from a relatively small increase in exercise. As you increase the level, the benefits improve too, but not in proportion. It is the law of diminishing returns.

It is even possible to exercise too much. World class endurance athletes are more prone to infectious diseases. In addition, they distort their dietary habits for maximum performance – to the detriment of their health.

So what is a reasonable compromise between what is desirable and what is possible?

Exercise Essentials

We can put together the foregoing paleo-anthropological argument with the studies and recommendations made by various authorities.

The recommended physical activity is :

    * 3 to 5 days per week of aerobic exercise at moderate to moderately high intensities.

    * 20 to 60 minutes each session.

That is the laconic specification. Let us look at what that means in practice.

'Moderate intensity aerobic exercise' is one that raises your heart rate to 40% of its maximum. Women, children and older men should aim to do this.

* Examples of moderate physical activity include:
  walking, cycling, playing basketball or volleyball, swimming, water aerobics, dancing fast, pushing a stroller, raking leaves, shovelling snow, washing or waxing a car, washing windows or floors, gardening, golf and tennis.

'Moderate to high intensity aerobic exercise' is one that raises your heart rate to 85% of its maximum. Able-bodied males should aim to do this.

* Examples of moderate to high intensity physical activity include:
  jogging/running, squash, hard swimming, vigorous cycling, manual labouring and weight training.

Don't forget that the above are minimums! Nothing to stop a women playing squash if she wants, or indeed a centenarian jogging 10 miles if he is fit enough.

In today's modern America, the problem is the opposite. Many children and young adults get out of breath just changing the channels on the remote control.

	Heart Rate: Beats per Minute		
Age	**40% Max.**	**85% Max.**	**Max.**
20	80	170	200
30	75	160	190
40	70	150	180
50	70*	145	170
60	65*	135	160
70	60*	125	150

*Many older people will have a resting pulse greater than this.

A word of warning. Anyone who has a history of smoking, is or has been severely overweight, is middle-aged or more, is under constant stress, has a family history of heart disease - should get a check up for potential problems. Advanced heart disease can have no symptoms. Even regular exercisers who fit into the above categories can be struck down without warning.

Jim Fixx, who wrote *The Complete Book Of Running* and thereby set off the jogging craze, was such a case. He had been a heavy smoker and had been very overweight. He had a poor family history, his father dying of a heart attack at the age of 43. Fixx quit smoking, lost 50 pounds of surplus weight and started running 60 to 70 miles a week. Everything was all right for 15 years. Then at the age of 52 he suffered a massive heart attack while running and died. His coronary arteries were hopelessly blocked. They were almost certainly far gone when he started his fitness regimen, but he didn't know - he had never had a check-up. And just being physically fit, contrary to what he thought, was not enough to stop his arteries getting worse. Rather, physical fitness is just one of the elements necessary to health and well being.

What about other forms of exercise? Callisthenics, muscle building, stretching and so on? Yes, they are all helpful. Indeed the recommendation is that everyone should be using stretching exercises at least three times a week. Elderly people are particularly recommended to do muscle building exercises and joint suppleness training every day. This will ensure that they arrest the loss of muscle mass and keep their joints flexible.

Savvy Exercising for Weight Loss

Many people exercise to lose weight. We can use a knowledge of our biochemistry to make sure this happens in the most efficient way.

When we exercise moderately (40% of max heart rate), then the source of energy that the body mostly uses comes from the triglyceride fats that are floating around in the blood stream. These are the fats that we want to burn! The body has to replace them from stores in the fat tissues.

If, however, we step up the exercise rate, then the body starts to prefer energy from carbohydrates stored in the liver, muscles and blood. The body will replace these later from what we eat.

The good news then, is that moderately intense exercise is better than high intensity exercise for fat reduction. This effect is particularly marked if no carbohydrates have been consumed before, during or after the exercise. So, go for your brisk, early morning walk on an empty stomach. Avoid all sugary drinks, and certainly don't eat any bad carbohydrates. If you must eat during this period, restrict it to the 'good' foods, some fruit for example. You won't feel hungry. Less conventionally, don't be inhibited by your cultural conditioning: it is quite possible to have a stir-fry or a mixed salad for breakfast.

Nutrition for Competitive Sports

Eating in order to obtain maximum performance is the domain of specialized sports nutrition. The only reason for broaching this topic here is to make an important point: sports nutrition has, as its main objective, the achievement of maximum *performance*.

───── ◆ ─────

Eating for maximum performance is rarely in harmony with nutrition for optimum health.

───── ◆ ─────

Take one example: 'carbohydrate loading'. This technique, to stoke up energy reserves before a race, makes extensive use of high glycemic index 'bad carbohydrates' that are consumed in a particular pattern over an extended number of days. To obtain maximum performance the technique is very good. But, this is exactly contrary to the principles of eating for good health.

This is a trade-off that is rarely explained to athletes: performance vs. long-term health.

Note too, that the 'savvy eating for weight loss' procedure explained earlier is the exact opposite to that prescribed for eating for endurance performance. For performance, athletes are recommended to consume high glycemic index foods (that is, *bad* carbohydrates) before, during and after the competition!

It is readily acknowledged by sports nutritionists that this causes hyperinsulinemia – and they know it wreaks havoc on arteries and scrambles hormonal responses. They know, too, that hyperinsulinemia locks up fat and makes it unavailable for burning by the muscles. This is a drawback. Nevertheless, the calculation they make is that this is the lesser of two evils - the greater energy surge from the bad carbohydrates outweighs the loss of energy generated from fat sources.

We have here an example of how food is used as a drug. A performance-enhancing drug for athletes. In various ways what and how you eat is having a drug-like effect on thousands of important bodily activities.

Lifestyle Practices

Not surprisingly, conventional wisdom is coming to the view that physical exercise should be more than just an episode on various days of the week. Physical exercise needs to be integrated into the everyday pattern of living.

First of all, try to develop hobbies, sports and interests that of themselves give you the base-load of exercise that you need. If you play golf one day a week, go dancing one day a week, do some gardening one day a week, and go swimming one day a week; then you are well on the way to being well-exercised. By all means go to aerobics, play tennis, jog round the block too.

Next, take every opportunity to work out those muscles as you go about your day. Why stress yourself to find a parking space right next to the shopping mall entrance? That only helps to raise stress hormones with all the damage that that does. Park at a comfortable distance away and walk those extra 100 yards! Walk up the stairs instead of taking the elevator. Carry the shopping instead of pushing the trolley.

Today, we are so spoiled for labor-saving devices that we have, perversely, to seek out labor intensive activities or make them up for ourselves. Push yourself constantly to stretch your body's physical capacity. Never take the easy way out when the opportunity is there to challenge your physical limits.

Chapter Twelve

Recipes and Structuring the Day

In Natural Eating the emphasis is on keeping meals simple and cooking as little as possible.

Vegetables

Vegetables should be used as fresh as possible. Store them in a cool, airy place like the vegetable rack of the refrigerator. Most vegetables can (and should) be eaten raw. Frozen vegetables are acceptable. Canned vegetables are acceptable in controlled situations where the convenience outweighs the nutritional drawbacks. Canned tomatoes, for example, are useful in 'quick-fix' dishes. AFD (Accelerated Freeze Dried) vegetables should be avoided.

Think big for your utensils. The quantities are at least double what you are used to. Get a really large salad bowl, wok and saucepan.

Raw Vegetables

Most vegetables can be eaten raw. Potato is an exception and cannot be eaten raw. It is indigestible and will create gas. Another clue to show that humans were not designed to eat potatoes.

Most legumes (lentils, beans etc.) are toxic until they are cooked. That is why it is necessary to boil them vigorously for the first ten minutes.

Raw vegetables may be eaten with a dip to add interest and taste. See the section on dips.

Cooked Vegetables

Unless the recipe specifies otherwise, vegetables should be lightly cooked and crunchy ('al dente' as the Italians say).

Stir-frying, the traditional Chinese method, uses no oil just a couple of teaspoons of water. Adopt this habit for healthiest results.

Frozen stir-fry vegetables are a good standby. They can be stir-fried, just as they come, in their own juices. No need to use a wok – just heat rapidly and stir constantly for 5 - 6 minutes in a large saucepan.

Sample Recipes

The Natural Eater is encouraged to avoid the formal meal structure of starter – main course – dessert. Nevertheless, there will be occasions when it is appropriate, or you want to put on a conventional format dinner party. For ease of reference, this segment is set out according to this plan.

Here follows a short selection of ideas for conforming Natural Eating dishes. It is assumed that most people already know how to prepare meat based dishes. For this reason there are none in this short collection. The reader is referred to the Natural Eating Recipe Book for a complete collection.

Notes

1. Units: the recipes are based on United States cookery measures. The metric figures are rounded conversions of these measures. It is possible, but not advised, to mix U.S. and metric measures in the same recipe.

2. Yeast extract: this is a good standby of vegetarian cookery and it figures in some of the following recipes. Yeast extract has an intense flavor, is relatively low in salt (12%) and, as a bonus, is full of B vitamins. It is difficult to find in some parts of the country but check with health food stores and quality supermarkets first.

   As a substitute, use vegetable stock cubes. These are usually loaded with salt (between 25% and 50%)and many other artificial flavor enhancers, so they are not the first choice.

   A blander alternative to either of these is vegetable broth, as sold in cartons like fresh fruit juice. Substitute the yeast extract and water of the recipe with the vegetable broth.

3. Stir-fry herbs: some recipes call for these. The basic mixture contains oregano, crushed bay leaves, basil and thyme. Make up your own mix using equal parts of these herbs, or find a proprietary product that conforms closely to this recipe.

Quick Fixes

When you are in a hurry it is good to have some simple food fixes up your sleeve. Here are a couple of ideas to set the tone. They trade convenience for some compromise in sophistication and nutritional rectitude.

Green Beans And Onion

Serves: 2

Method

* In the saucepan, sauté the frozen onion until defrosted and tender, and there is no liquid left.

* Add the oil and bring up to frying heat quickly.

* Add the green beans and continue to sauté for 5 minutes.

* Add the tomato paste and herbs.

* Stir and cook for 2 more minutes.

Ingredients:

* 1 lb. (455 g.) green beans, cut, frozen

* 8 oz. (225 g.) onions, chopped, frozen

* 4 oz. (115 g.) tomato paste

* 4 tsp. (20 g.) stir fry herbs, (see Note 3)

* 1 tbs. (15 ml.) canola oil

Comment

This meal can be prepared very quickly and simply. The onions and beans are both 'good' vegetables. If you are slimming avoid the use of oil. Simply sauté the onions in their own juices. Learn to use herbs to provide exciting flavors.

Cauliflower Cheese

Serves: 2

Method

* Clean the cauliflower head of extraneous leaves and rinse it thoroughly.

* Boil the whole head until cooked lightly (about 5 minutes). Better to steam if you have the time (about 15 minutes.)

* Drain the head and set to one side on a large plate.

* Cut the cheese into small cubes and put into a microwave-proof bowl.

* Melt the cheese in a microwave oven. (Turn occasionally and use several 20 second bursts until the cheese is melted through - about 80 seconds.)

* Pour the melted cheese uniformly over the cauliflower head.

Ingredients:

* 1 large head, 18 oz. (510 g.) cauliflower

* 6 oz. (170 g.) cheddar cheese, sharp

Comment:

Cheese? Yes, 3 oz. of cheese two to three times a week is quite admissible from a health point of view provided you are keeping up the high consumption of vegetation.

Choose a good sharp whole cheese whose flavor spreads thinly. You might have to experiment with different makes of cheddar to find one that melts well without separation. Low fat cheese does not melt well and is not recommended. Cheese can be an allergen, so sensitive people should be alert to this possibility.

The ratio of vegetable (and alkaline) food to high density (and acid) cheese is reasonable at 3 to 1. Cauliflower is a SuperVeg. Eat often.

Starters

Salad Dressings

Salad dressings should be free of dairy products except, on occasion, fat-free yogurt (no cream, butter, cheese etc.) and free of starches, particularly corn-flour, thickeners and sugars. It is possible to find good ready-made salad dressings which conform to this specification but read the fine print.

Make up your own basic dressing (see following recipe) in quantity and keep it in the refrigerator.

Basic Salad Dressing

Main course: serves: 2, side dish: serves: 4

Method:

* Beat the oil and salt together in the salad bowl until the salt dissolves.

* Add the other ingredients and whisk to a creamy texture with a fork.

Ingredients:

* 4 tbs. (60 ml.) virgin canola oil
* 1 tbs. (15 ml.) lemon juice
* 1 tbs. (15 ml.) tomato juice, unsalted
* 1/4 tsp. salt
* 1 pinch pepper
* 3 cloves garlic, crushed

Comment:

Canola oil is a good basic oil. More expensive but flavorful alternatives are flax and walnut oil. (Olive oil is OK too, but it is just empty calories.) Definitely do not use any other kind of oil.

Provençale Salad

Serves: 4

Method:

* Slice the raw zucchini into very fine slices.

* Cut the bell peppers into small strips and the tomatoes in slices.

* Remove and discard the seeds from the tomatoes.

* Cut the spring onions, including healthy green stems, into small slices.

* Arrange the zucchini in a bottom layer and dust lightly with salt and pepper.

* Add the bell peppers in a decorative arrangement.

* Decorate the surface with the tomato and dust lightly with salt and pepper.

* Trickle in some basic salad dressing. Sprinkle the basil and parsley

* Add the olives.

Ingredients:

* 1 yellow bell pepper
* 1 red bell pepper
* 1 green pepper
* 3 zucchini
* 3 tomatoes
* 6 spring onions
* 16 olives, black, pitted
* basic salad dressing
* chopped basil
* chopped parsley
* salt and pepper

Comment:

On two occasions the recipe calls for a light dusting with salt. It means just that, no more than a pinch or two on each occasion.

Lentil Soup

serves: 4

Method:

* Dissolve the yeast extract in the hot water and put in a 1 gallon saucepan.

* Add the lentils, garlic, tomatoes, cloves and bay leaves.

* Bring rapidly to the boil and simmer for 15 minutes

* Chop the vegetables coarsely as necessary and add to saucepan.

* Simmer for a further 15 minutes.

* Remove from saucepan and blend in a mixer to a hearty consistency.

* Serve.

Ingredients:

* 1 lb. (455 g.) green lentils.

* 1 lb. (455 g.) leeks, frozen

* 8 oz. (225 g.) baby carrots

* 8 oz. (225 g.) celery

* 1 tin, 16 oz. (455 g.) tomatoes, chopped

* 2 tsp. (10 ml.) yeast extract (see note 2)

* 2 cloves garlic, crushed

* 2 cloves

* 2 bay leaves

* 1 cup (225 ml.) hot water

Comment:

Note the high proportion of vegetables to lentils (a high protein food). This is a good vegetation/protein ratio. It has the further advantage of limiting any disagreeable flatulence effects from the lentils. The high glycemic carrots are well diluted by the other ingredients.

Main Course

Roasted Summer Vegetables

Serves: 4 to 6

Method:

* Halve the onions through the root, leaving the root intact. Peel them and cut each half in two lengthwise to give 4 pieces. Precook the onions by steaming for 5 minutes.

* Halve and seed the peppers, removing the stalks and any white membrane. Cut each pepper into quarters.

* Carefully cut the garlic heads in half through the equator.

* Cut the eggplants in half lengthwise.

Ingredients:

* 2 medium onions
* 2 medium red bell peppers
* 2 large heads garlic
* 2 eggplants, Japanese
* 2 tomatoes
* 1 squash
* 2 zucchini (optional)
* 8 button mushrooms (optional)
* 4 fl. oz. (110 ml.) olive oil
* 4 sprigs fresh (or dried) thyme
* black pepper, fresh
* coarse salt, frugal

* Cut the tomatoes in half through the equator.

* Cut the squash lengthwise into 8 slices.

* Halve or quarter the zucchini.

* Place all these vegetables in a roasting tin. Drizzle the olive oil and sprinkle the thyme, salt and pepper over all.

* Roast in a preheated oven at 400°F (200°C) for about 35 minutes, turning the vegetables twice. They should be tender and browning, but not disintegrating. The garlic should be golden and soft.

Comment:

This is a hearty, varied vegetable dish. It is quite filling, and can easily serve as a complete meal in itself. It uses a lot of oil. Slimmers should eat frugally.

Lentils and Nut Loaf

Serves: 4 - 6

Method:

* Drain the lentils.

* Sauté the onions with the oil in a small saucepan very briefly. When they start to stick, add a little water and cook them, covered, on low heat. From time to time, as they dry out, add a little more water. Cook until the onions have a very soft consistency, they should not be at all browned.

* Add the soy sauce to the onions and mix in the lentils and nuts.

* Beat the eggs, add the remaining ingredients and blend into the lentil mixture.

Ingredients:

* 1 can (14 oz., 400 g.) lentils, cooked

* 2 medium (9 oz., 250 g.) onions, white, finely diced to lentil size

* 5 oz. (145 g.) walnuts, raw, roughly ground in a blender

* 3 eggs

* 1 tbs. (15 ml.) canola oil

* 1 tbs. (15 ml.) soy sauce[1]

* 1 clove garlic, crushed

* 5 leaves sage, fresh, chopped finely

* 1 tsp. thyme, fresh or dried

* 2 tsp. parsley, fresh, chopped (optional)

* pepper

* Place the mixture into a 1½ lb. (680 g.) small oiled loaf tin.

* Bake at 375°F (190°C) for 20 to 25 mins.

* Turn out of the tin and serve, in thick slices, hot or cold.

Comment:

This is a rich, high protein dish. One thick slice makes a good portion as a side dish. It can be served with a light tomato sauce.

---

1. A better alternative, if you have it, is 1tsp. (5ml.) yeast extract dissolved in 1tbs. (15ml) hot water.

Vegetable Curry

Serves: 6

Method:

* Heat the oil in the saucepan and add the onion.

* Cook gently until the onion is soft, stirring from time to time. Add a little water as necessary.

* Add the curry powder, garlic and sauté briefly.

* Add the tomatoes, stirring the while.

* Add the vegetable broth, carrots and potatoes.

* Bring to the boil and cook, covered, for 15 - 20 minutes (according to the quality of the potatoes and carrots).

* Add the cauliflower florets and cashews.

* Cook for another 5 minutes.

* Add the green bell pepper.

* Cook for another 10 minutes. (The bell pepper should still look green at the end.)

Ingredients:

* 16 oz. (455 g.) onions, chopped
* 2 tbs. (30 ml.) canola or olive oil
* 4 tbs. curry powder, Madras (medium)
* 4 cloves garlic, crushed
* 28 oz. (800 g.) tomatoes, canned, chopped
* 1 cup (225 ml.) vegetable broth
* 16 oz. (455 g.) potatoes, peeled, diced
* 10 oz. (280 g.) carrots, diced
* 16 oz. (455 g.) cauliflower florets
* 4 tbs. cashews, raw, chopped
* 2 (12 oz., 340 g.) green bell peppers, seeded and diced.

Comment:

Curried dishes provide an interesting variation on more familiar dishes.

Be careful not to make them too hot. Beware of the irritation effect on intestines and mucus membranes. Sensitive people should keep the curry mild and eat modestly.

Potatoes? This recipe makes a point: that by *diluting bad* carbohydrate (here 1 lb.) with plentiful (here 5 lb.) *favourable* carbohydrates, the overall result is acceptable. See Appendix 1, Glycemic Indexes, Mixed Carbohydrates.

Sauces/Dips

Dips should be free of dairy products and starches, particularly corn-flour, thickeners and sugars. It is possible to find good ready-made sauce/dips such as salsa, guacamole and low fat hummus which conform to this specification but read the fine print! You will only find them in the chilled shelves of shops catering to the quality market.

Here we give the recipes of two dips that you can make for yourself.

Black Olive Tapenade[2]

Method:

* Drain the olives and set aside the liquid.

* Blend all the ingredients together, adding the liquid from the olives until a creamy consistency is obtained.

Ingredients:

* 2 cans (24 oz., 680 mg.) olives, black, pitted
* 10 tbs. (150 ml.) liquid from olives
* 4 tbs. (60 ml.) olive oil
* 1/2 oz. (15 g.) garlic
* 2 tsp. (10 ml.) vinegar, red wine
* 2 tbs. (30 g.) canned capers
* 2 tsp. (10 ml.) lemon juice
* 2 tsp. thyme
* 1/4 tsp. pepper

Comment:

This sauce is good both served as a sauce for whole-wheat spaghetti and as a raw vegetable dip. Experiment with different amounts of the liquid to obtain the consistency desired. Thicker is best as a dip, thinner as a sauce.

2. Traditional sauce from Provence in the South of France.

Mexican Dip

Method:

* Soak and cook the kidney beans in accordance with the instructions on the packet.

* Put all the ingredients into a food processor or blender and process until it is smooth.

* Serve as a dip for raw vegetables, etc.

Ingredients:

* 8 oz. (225 g.) dry weight, red kidney beans

* 3 (21 oz., 600 g.) red bell peppers, seeded

* 8 oz. (1 can, 225 ml.) tomato juice, unsalted

* 1 tbs. (15 ml.) canola oil

* 1 tbs. (15 ml.) chili sauce, to taste

* 1 tbs. (15 ml.) yeast extract. (see Note 2)

Comment:

This is a hearty, healthy, strong tasting dip, free of dairy products and bad fats.

By utilizing slightly less tomato juice, the dip takes on the consistency of a pâté and can then be served as a high protein side dish.

Desserts

Chocolate Mousse

Serves: 4

Method:

* Grate only the colored part of the orange and set aside.

* Carefully break the eggs and separate the yolk from the white.

* Break the chocolate into small pieces and put into a microwave-proof bowl.

* Add the rum, instant coffee and the water.

* Melt the mixture in a microwave, checking and stirring frequently. Avoid overheating.

Ingredients:

* 7 oz. (200 g.) dark, bitter chocolate with minimum 70% cocoa solids (see comment)

* 4 eggs

* 1 tbs. (15 g.) fructose

* 1 orange (preferably organic)

* 4 tbs. (60 ml.) dark, flavorful rum

* 2 tsp. (10 g.) instant coffee (can be decaffeinated) in 3 tbs. (45 ml.) hot water

* 4 tbs. (60 ml.) water

* Take the yolks and the fructose and mix to creamy texture.

* Add half the grated orange peel to the mixture.

* Beat the egg whites with a pinch of salt until very stiff.

* Add the yolk/sugar mixture to the chocolate mixture.

* Blend to a smooth consistency.

* Add the egg-whites progressively to the mixture, stirring carefully to obtain a smooth consistency.

* Put the mixture into a dessert bowl.

* Sprinkle the remaining orange peel gratings over the top.

* Conserve in a refrigerator for a minimum of 5 hours. (Ideally, for full flavor, make the mousse the day before consumption.)

Comment:

If you cannot find 70% chocolate, then instead use 4 oz. (115 g.) bittersweet chocolate with a minimum of 50% cocoa solids and 3 oz. (85 g.) unsweetened baking chocolate, 100% cocoa solids.

This dish is an interesting example of how a superb dessert can be made from high density chocolate and fructose. The eggs make this a protein-dominated dessert, so it goes best after a protein meal. There is some debate as to whether the alcohol in the rum sterilizes the uncooked eggs. It is advisable to observe the usual precautions regarding consumption by vulnerable people (the elderly, the very young, pregnant women and the immune-compromised).

Baked Apple Dessert

Serves: 4

Method:

* Core the apples. Score the skin around the equator.

* Stuff the cores with the dried fruit, pressing in firmly.

* Put into microwave-proof dish and loosely cover with grease-proof paper.

* Microwave on full power for about 5 minutes, or until the apples are soft but not collapsed.

* Sprinkle with cinnamon and serve.

Ingredients:

* 4 baking apples (8 oz., 225 g. each)

* 3 oz. (85 g.) mixed dried fruit

* 1 tsp. cinnamon.

Comment:

This dish also makes a nice snack at any time.

Food Combining:

Even though this is a fruit, and it is to be eaten at the end of a meal, this should not present any problems. Cooking the apple will have destroyed many enzymes, including those that could give a digestive difficulty.

Carbohydrate Status:

This dish is a low density, borderline carbohydrate. One apple per person is plenty and, if eaten at the end of a meal free of bad carbohydrates, then this dish will be quite safe.

Nutritional Status:

The apple is slightly the worse for cooking - but it is still a good dish.

Note that there is no sugar called for, nor needed.

Beverage

Hot cocoa drink

serves: 1

Method:

* Put the cocoa powder into a mug.

* Add milk (if used) and stir well, or add small amount of hot water as necessary to mix.

* Pour on boiling water, stirring well.

* Allow the drink to cool to drinking temperature.

* Add the aspartame to taste.

Ingredients:

* 2 tsp. pure cocoa powder.

* 2 tsp. (10 ml.) milk (optional)

* 12 oz. (340 ml.) boiling water.

* Aspartame to taste

Comment:

This is a safe cocoa drink. Definitely avoid the multitude of proprietary "hot chocolate" drinks. Mostly they are full of sugars, fillers, substitutes and junk ingredients.

Milk? Not the ideal, but for otherwise healthy people, the consumption of 2 tsp. of milk a couple of times a day is not significant.

Aspartame? As explained earlier, the use of artificial sweeteners as a replacement for sugar, is much the lesser of two evils. Aspartame loses its sweetening power with high heat. By waiting until the drink is cooler less Aspartame needs to be used.

Sample Daily Eating Patterns

There is an infinity of ways of putting together a feeding pattern for the day. Four schedules of daily eating patterns are given on the following pages. (A longer regimen is given in the Natural Eating Manual.) These schedules are just examples to give an idea of the range and variety possible. Don't feel that you have to follow any one of them slavishly. Use your imagination to substitute and experiment.

Pattern #1 No Starch, Work Day, Restaurant Dinner					
Time	**Foodstuff**	**amount**	**Quantity oz.**	**gram**	**Comments**
Morning Start					
07.30	melon, honeydew	1 slice	4.0	115	This is a high G.I.[3] but low density fruit[4]
08.30	apricots	4 count	7.0	200	Washed for eating on the journey to work
Mid-morning					
10.00	pears	3 count	20.0	570	Washed, cored and cut into morsels asnecessary and brought to eat
	apple, large	2 count	12.0	340	at work
Canteen Lunch					
12.30	lettuce		4.0	115	Mixed Salad
	cucumber		4.0	115	
	radish		2.0	55	
	tomato		4.0	115	
	broccoli		2.0	55	Stir-fry: ask for double portion of vegetables
	bamboo shoots		3.0	85	Optionally: If the rice is whole-meal (brown) a portion of that will be all right
	bok choi		3.0	85	
	carrots		2.0	55	
	celery		4.0	115	
	water chestnuts		4.0	115	
	canola oil	1 tbs.	0.5	15	

3 G.I. = Glycemic Index
4 This quantity yields 2tsp. of sucrose. Safe for healthy people, but don't eat more.

Time	Foodstuff		Quantity		Comments
		amount	oz.	gram	

Pattern #1
No Starch, Work Day, Restaurant Dinner

Time	Foodstuff	amount	oz.	gram	Comments
Afternoon Break					
16.00	guacamole		3.5	100	Brought to work in lunch box
	cauliflower, raw		6.1	175	
Dinner Time					
19.00					**Pre-dinner Cocktail**[5]
	cashew nuts		1.0	30	Protein nibbles. Avoid the chips
	olives		1.0	30	Oily nibble
	tomato juice	1 glass	3.5	100	
20.00					**Restaurant Dinner**[6]
	mushrooms		2.0	55	Starter, mushrooms in olive oil
	olive oil		0.5	15	Avoid mopping up excess oil
	peas		1.0	30	Main Course
	asparagus[7]		2.0	55	
	green beans[7]		3.0	85	
	salmon, grilled		4.0	115	Half portion[8] - the rest is for the doggy bag
	wine, red	1 glass	3.5	100	Just the one glass
Total Weight			**6.6 lb.**	**3.0 kg.**	**Weights are net (as eaten)**

5 Ask the waiter to take away the bad carbohydrate nibbles and to bring nuts and olives. (This is an upmarket restaurant.)
6 Take care not to eat the warm rolls that come with the meal.
7 These vegetables have been negotiated with the waiter as a substitute for the wild rice that normally accompanies the salmon dish.
8 This is to keep the protein rush under control. 4 oz. of fish is plenty at one sitting.

		Pattern #2			
		All Vegetable Day			
Comment: This day is based entirely on vegetables. This represents an extreme. It is good to do from time to time but there is no obligation. The idea is to demonstrate here how it can be done.					

Time	Foodstuff	Quantity			Comments
		amount	oz.	gram	
Morning start					
08.00	fresh bean shoots, stir fried.	1 bag	12.0	340	Start the morning with a stir-fry
	olive oil	(1 tsp.)	0.2	6	Just enough to cover the pan
09.00	peas in pod[9]	16 oz.	6.0	170	Snacks - eaten throughout the day
	almonds raw		3.0	85	Mid-morning snack
11.00	vegetable curry		16.0	455	*See recipe*
Lunch-time					
13.00	tomatoes, fresh		16.0	455	Large tomato salad
	spring onion		1.0	30	
	beetroot		5.0	145	(Low density, borderline G.I.)
Mid-afternoon snack					
15.30	mixed leaf salad	1 pack	8.0	225	
	standard dressing (recipes)	2 tbs.	1.0	30	
Dinner-time					
18.30	roasted summer vegetables		16.0	455	*See recipe*
Supper-time					
21.00	broccoli, steamed		12.0	340	Supper if required
	walnut oil[10]	1 tbs.	0.5	15	
22.00	cocoa drink, mug	1 tbs.	0.5	15	*See recipe*
Weight			**6.1 lb.**	**2.7 kg.**	**Weights are net (as eaten)**

9 It is good to buy peas in pod when in season. They are practical too for taking on trips.
10 Use omega 3 oils like canola (best) and walnut or flax for cold dressings

Time	Foodstuff	amount	Quantity oz.	gram	Comments
		Pattern #3 Out and About			
Morning of Fruit Eating					
08.15	grapefruit	2	16.0	455	Favorable G.I. fruit
09.00	apple	3 count	18.0	510	Cored, sliced and packed in zip-lock bag to carry out and about
10.00	cherries		16.0	455	Washed and packed in zip-lock bag
11.30	strawberries	punnet	8.0	225	Washed and packed in zip-lock bag
Packed Lunch					
13.00					
	pita bread pocket[11]	1 round	2.0	55	Makes a good sandwich[12]
	alfalfa sprouts	punnet	4.0	115	
Mid-afternoon Snack					
(Fast Food Salad Bar) Use no salad dressing. Ask for the oil and vinegar cruet. If you are well organized, bring your own salad dressing. This is a big salad. Each portion takes up a polystyrene plate. Go back to the bar as often as it takes.					
16.00	broccoli, raw		3.5	100	
	cucumber		3.5	100	
	lettuce		3.5	100	
	tomatoes		3.5	100	
	coleslaw		3.5	100	
	pickled beets		3.5	100	Borderline G.I. This modest quantity is fine for healthy people
	vinaigrette	2 tbs.	1.0	30	Take care to consume no more than this
Evening Light Meal					
18.30	omelet[13], plain	2 eggs	3.5	100	
	baby spinach salad	1/2 pack	3.5	100	
	basic salad dressing 1 tbs.		0.5	15	
Supper - protein oriented					
20.30	cheese, brie[14]	nibble	1.0	30	Gourmet nibble to enjoy with the tomato
	tomatoes	one	3.5	100	
	wine, red	1 glass	3.5	100	
Total Weight			6.3 lb.	2.9 kg.	Weights are net (as eaten)

11 Whole wheat Pita bread. Made only from whole wheat, water, yeast and possibly salt
12 The Pita round sliced in half and each half opened up to make a pocket. It is capable of holding a very high volume of filling. This keeps the proportion of bread to vegetable at a suitably low figure.
13 Can substitute, say, lentil dish (see recipes)
14 Can substitute 1 oz nuts - like cashews, brazil, almonds, walnuts.

Pattern #4
All Fruit Day

Comment:

This is an extreme case which is not obligatory! However it is healthful to have an all fruit day, say, once a month. This allows the body to have a respite from having to treat a constant input of toxin-creating foodstuffs and to eliminate any build-up. Eating this way gives the full complement of macro- and micro-nutrients, with the possible exception of protein.

There is nothing particular about the selection of fruits. It is just as wide a variety as possible, given availability in the market.

Note that fruit is eaten at will throughout the day. There is nothing special about the individual weights or the times. Just eat each time you feel hungry. Note also the great weight consumed, about 11 pounds. Since the quantities are so large, it is possible to over-consume high G.I. fruits. Take care to manage this aspect.

This large volume even supplies 40 g. of protein. This is quite a surprising and respectable quantity for a day that has no 'protein-rich' food in it. Even so, 40 g/day is on the low side for a full size adult, so it is not recommended that anyone should eat every day like this.

Time	Foodstuff	amount	Quantity oz.	gram	Comments
9.00	pears	2 count	12	340	
9.30	grapes	1 bunch	12	340	borderline G.I.
10.00	plums	10 count	16	455	
11.00	fresh fig	4 count	12	340	borderline G.I.
13.00	tomatoes[15]	4 count	18	510	
14.30	grapefruit	3 count	24	680	
17.00	strawberries	punnet	14	395	
18.30	cherries		16	455	
	apricots	10 count	16	455	
	kiwi fruit	3 count	12	340	
20.30	apples	3 large	16	455	
Total Weight			**11.0 lb.**	**5.0 kg.**	**Weights are net (as eaten)**

---

15 Tomato is technically a fruit, but is usually thought of, and can be consumed as, a vegetable too.

a p p e n d i x   o n e

Tables

Good Foods

This is a collection of the foods that are soundly located in the Natural Eating profile. The first table, foods to be eaten without restriction, are basically plant foods, analogous to those eaten copiously by our Pleistocene ancestors. Just like our Pleistocene ancestors, there are other foods that would have been available in controlled quantities. These are represented in table 2. In the modern world there is a small difference – we have to exercise self-discipline to limit the amounts eaten.

For that reason, in Table 2, there are portion sizes indicated. You don't have to follow them slavishly – use them as a guide. After all, the greater your ideal weight, the greater will be your food needs. That is, a 6'-3" lean person will have significantly greater food needs than a 5'-0" lean person. Read table 2 in conjunction with the recommendations in Chapter Ten, *The Ten Steps to Success.*

Table 1 Examples of **Good Foods to be Eaten in Bulk** Eat as much as you like a minimum of 4 lb. to 6 lb. per day from this list		
Vegetables	**Fruits fresh**	**Salads**
artichoke	apple	alfalfa sprouts
asparagus	apricot	bean sprouts
aubergine (egg plant)	blackberry	bell pepper - all varieties
bok choy	cherry	broccoli
broccoli	grapefruit	cabbage
brussels sprouts	orange	cauliflower
cabbage	peach	celery
cauliflower	pear	coleslaw
celeriac	plum - all varieties	cress
chicory	raspberry	cucumber
fennel	strawberry	endive
french beans	tomato	escarole
green beans	nectarine	garlic
kale		lettuce - all varieties
kohl rabi		mushroom - all varieties
leeks		onion - all varieties
okra		palm heart
peas, sugar snap	**Herbs & Spices**[1]	radish
spinach		spinach
swiss chard		spring onion
tomato, raw		tomato - all varieties
turnip		water chestnut
vegetable marrow		watercress
zucchini		

1 All herbs and spices are good to use copiously with the exception of hot spices like chilli, mustard, curry and pepper. These should be used frugally.

Table 2
Examples of
Good Foods to be Eaten in Controlled Quantities
portion size as noted
Read in Conjunction with Chapter Ten

Pastas (dry weight)		**Legumes (dry weight)**		**Fish**	
spaghetti, whole-wheat	4 oz.	beans[2]	3 oz.	herring, canned, oil	2 oz.
Cereals (dry weight)		lentils	3 oz.	lobster, crab	2 oz.
oatmeal	2 oz.	hummus	2 oz.	mackerel	3 oz.
barley; rye kernels	4 oz.	soy protein & products	2 oz.	salmon	3 oz.
rye kernel bread, slices[3]	2	peas	6 oz.	sardine, in water	3 oz.
		baked beans	6 oz.	tuna	3 oz.
Vegetables		**Fruits**		**Nuts**	
avocado, 1 item	8 oz.	banana, ripe	3 oz.	almonds	2 oz.
marrowfat peas	4 oz.	banana, green	6 oz.	brazil nut	2 oz.
carrots, raw	8 oz.	grapes	6 oz.	cashew	2 oz.
guacamole[4]	4 oz.	kiwi	6 oz.	chestnut	3 oz.
potato, new, waxy, boiled	6 oz.	mango	6 oz.	cob, hazel nut	2 oz.
beets	4 oz.	melon	6 oz.	walnut	2 oz.
yam	6 oz.	papaya	4 oz.		
		pineapple	4 oz.		
		watermelon	6 oz.		
				Poultry	
				chicken breast, skinless	3 oz.
				turkey breast, skinless	3 oz.
		Sugar/confectionery		**Eggs & Products**	
		fructose	4 tsp.	egg substitute	3 oz
		dark chocolate[5]	2 oz.	eggs, chicken	2

Accessories (can be added to above)

Beverages *per day*		**Fats and Oils** *per day*		**Condiments**	
tea, black , bag	3	canola oil, or	2 tbs.	canola mayonnaise	2 tbs.
tea, green , bag	3	canola lite spread, or,	2 tbs.	fresh salsa sauce	2 tbs.
cocoa[6]	4 tsp.	flax oil, or	2 tbs.	ketchup	2 tbs.
wine, dry, glass	two	walnut oil	2 tbs.	pepper	
coffee, instant	3 tsp.	olive oil	1 tbs.	Worcester sauce	2 tbs.
				mustard - limit	

2 Beans: pinto, haricot/navy, kidney, lima, butter, black, soy, garbanzo (chick-pea). Not broad beans.
3 Rye kernel bread. It must be wheat flour-free (read the fine print) and will have some 50% as integral kernels. It is often sold at deli counters and has the size and density of a brick.
4 Guacamole is a preparation of pureed avocado seasoned with condiments.
5 Chocolate with a low sugar content. It is dark and bitter. The ingredient list will rank cocoa solids first.
6 Use only pure cocoa powder. 'Hot chocolate' drinks are usually full of nasties and fillers.

Glycemic Indexes

There are three tables that follow, giving glycemic indexes for some foodstuffs selected from The Natural Eating Manual. It is important to understand how to interpret them.

Glycemic index (G.I.) is measured by feeding the foodstuff being studied to volunteers, and measuring the rise and fall in their blood sugar over time. There are several variables that can give rise to a range of results:

- If eight (say) volunteers are tested simultaneously for a particular foodstuff, each person will react slightly differently. The G.I. will be the average for the eight results.

- Different varieties of a species usually have a different G.I. Both potatoes and rice have widely differing G.I.s according to the variety. In the tables presented here, the averages have been taken. For details by variety, refer to the Natural Eating Manual.

- The amount of cooking makes a difference. In general the more a carbohydrate is cooked, the more its structure is broken down and the higher its G.I.

- The amount of processing makes a difference. For example, oats are usually rolled in the factory prior to being sold as oatmeal or as a muesli ingredient. The more they are rolled the higher their G.I. Fast cooking oats have had the most pre-treatment and have the highest G.I.

- The degree of maturity can make a difference. Fruits, notably bananas, have higher G.I.'s the riper they are.

So all the G.I.'s are *averages*. The range of variation around the average can be great or little. It is impossible to be very precise about the G.I. of the particular carbohydrate that you are about to put into your mouth. Nevertheless, the ranking of each foodstuff relative to others holds very well. That is why the full range of foodstuffs is separated into *bad*, *borderline* and *favorable* carbohydrates.

For the foregoing reasons, the choice of where the separation falls is somewhat arbitrary. The important point is that *bad* carbohydrate corresponds closely with foodstuffs that we were never designed to eat and *favorable* carbohydrates correlate closely with the foods that we are designed to eat.

Notice also that a distinction is made between 'high density', 'medium density' and 'low density' carbohydrates. The significance is this: the quantity of carbohydrate that you eat at a sitting makes a difference. Consuming just one cornflake is hardly likely to make your blood sugar career out of control! So how many cornflakes does it take? Just one bowl? Or a bowl of cornflakes plus a waffle and maple syrup?

You, as an individual, will have your own threshold. This threshold is reached much faster the denser the carbohydrate. For example, carrots have a high glycemic index, especially when cooked. However, carrots are mostly water. Thus a healthy person (non-diabetic) has to eat a lot of them (about 16 oz.) to get the effect. 16 oz. of carrots contain about 1 tablespoon of sugar.

Carrots therefore make Table 2, Good Foods to be Eaten in Controlled Quantities. For example an 8 oz. pack of ready-to-eat raw baby carrots should be well tolerated. On the other hand, watch out for the fresh carrot juice in cartons. This is a danger. It has a higher glycemic index and it is only too easy to down a pint (16 oz.) in one go.

Also note that as you get older your body's ability to cope with blood-sugar stress gets lower. This is how 'middle age spread' creeps up unawares. You might have changed nothing in your lifestyle but suddenly you are putting on weight. Your threshold has dropped past the point where your body can cope with your eating habits.

———————— ◆ ————————

In middle age, your threshold resistance to high glycemic foods has dropped below the point where your body can cope with your eating habits.

———————— ◆ ————————

What about mixed meals? Various studies have shown that it doesn't change the basic calculation. The bun from the hamburger has much the same blood-sugar effect whether eaten on its own or with the meat patty.

When you mix carbohydrates, the combined G.I is the resultant of the individual weighted G.I.'s. Take an easy example: 8 oz. of baked potato (G.I. = 85) eaten with 4 oz. of green peas (G.I. = 45). The combined G.I. of this meal is 8 x 85 + 4 x 45 divided by 8 + 4. This calculates out to a combined G.I. for the meal of about 70. This shows how, by concurrently eating a lower G.I. food, it reduces the 'spike' of a high G.I. food. Even so, in this particular example, this mixed meal still lies within the *bad* carbohydrate category.

This is an example of how it is possible to use knowledge of G.I. mechanisms to steer a way through the minefield of *bad* carbohydrates. This topic, including a full list of glycemic indexes, is treated in greater detail in The Natural Eating Manual.

Table 3
Examples of
Bad Carbohydrates
indices 65 to 110
Insulin Reaction Potentially Dangerous to Health

High Density - 40% to 100% Carbohydrate

Sugars & Confectionery	Starches (Bakery)	Starches (Cereals)
100 glucose	95 French baguette	85 cornflakes
90 jam	70 muffin	80 rice cereal
80 jelly beans	70 corn chips	75 rice, low amylose
70 high fructose corn syrup	70 bagel, white	75 breakfast cereals (most)
70 honey	70 water crackers	70 shredded wheat
70 candy bar	70 bread, whole-wheat	70 gnocchi
65 brown sugar	70 bread, wheat, white	
65 white sugar	65 shortbread	
65 maple syrup		

Medium Density - 15% to 40% Carbohydrate

Starches (Vegetable)	Starches (Bakery)	Starches (Cereals)
85 baked potato	75 waffles	90 rice, instant, brown
70 french fries	70 croissant, French	90 rice pasta,

Low Density - Under 15% Carbohydrate

Starches (Vegetable)	Fruits
85 carrots, *cooked*	70 melon
75 pumpkin	70 watermelon
80 potato, micro-waved	65 pineapple
70 potato, boiled	
70 potato, mashed	

Drinks

90 cola, regular
70 orange soda

Table 4
Examples of
Borderline Carbohydrates
indices 40 to 60
Insulin Reaction Potentially Undermining to Health

High density - 40% to 100% Carbohydrate

Sugars & Confectionery	Starches (Bakery)	Starches (Cereals)
60 muesli bar	60 pita bread, white	60 muesli
Fruits	60 pizza - cheese	60 popcorn
65 *dried* fruit, generally	45 rye kernel bread	55 sweetcorn
65 raisins, dates, figs		40 spaghetti, white
60 sultanas		

Medium Density – 15% to 40% Carbohydrate

Fruit & Fruit Products	Starch (Vegetable)	Starches (Cereals)
60 banana, ripe	50 sweet potato	60 rice, white
55 mango	50 potato chips (crisps)	60 rice, wild
45 banana, green	**Legumes**	55 rice, brown
	50 lentils, green canned	55 spaghetti, durum
	50 kidney beans, canned	45 macaroni

Low Density - Under 15% Carbohydrate

Fruit & Fruit Products	Starch (Vegetable)	Starches (Cereals)
60 papaya	60 beets (beetroot)	60 porridge, regular
50 orange juice	60 potato, new	55 oatmeal[7]
50 kiwi fruit	50 carrot, raw	
45 grapes	**Legumes**	
40 orange	45 baked beans, canned	
40 peach, fresh	45 peas, green	

7 Made with water.

Table 5
Examples of
Favorable Carbohydrates
indices 0 to 35
Insulin Reaction Not Threatening to Health

High and Medium Density Carbohydrates
Eat in Controlled Quantities

Sugars	Vegetable Protein	Starches (Cereal)
25 chocolate, *80% cocoa solids*	35 haricot/navy beans	35 rye, whole kernel
20 fructose	30 lentils	35 spaghetti, wholemeal
Fruits	30 garbanzo (chick pea)	30 barley, pearled
15 avocado	20 soy beans	
	15 almond	
	15 walnut	

Low Density - under 15% carbohydrate
Unrestricted

Fruits	Vegetables	Vegetables
35 apple	15 asparagus	15 alfalfa sprouts
35 blackberries	15 broccoli	15 bell pepper - all varieties
35 pear	15 brussels sprouts	15 celery
35 plums	15 cabbage	15 cucumber
35 raspberries	15 cauliflower	15 lettuce - all varieties
35 strawberries	15 green beans	15 mushroom - all varieties
30 apricots	15 leeks	15 onion - all varieties
25 cherries	15 peas, sugar snap	15 radish
25 grapefruit	15 spinach	15 tomato
	15 zucchini	
	15 bell pepper - all varieties	

Bibliography

There are thousands of scientific articles published every year in peer-review journals. Many more appear in symposium reports and in accredited scientific journals and magazines. This rich resource has been extensively exploited in the development of the Natural Eating precepts. It is quite impossible to mention all those that have been influential. The following list of references contains a sample selection. They are chiefly from peer-review journals. For the sake of brevity sometimes the condensed, or paraphrased version of the title has been used. Also for the sake of brevity, the names of the journals have been reduced to an acronym. The concordance is to be found at the end of the bibliography.

In a similar vein, where there are references to published books and reports, a truncated reference is given, followed by a (P). The full publishing details will likewise be found at the end of the bibliography.

Bone Health/Calcium
Adams et al; Vitamin D Bone Intoxication; AIM; 1997; 127; 203-306
Allen et al; Protein Induced Hypercalciuria - a Longer Term Study; AJCN; 1979 Apr, 32:4, 741-9
Barzel et al; Excess Dietary Protein can Adversely Affect Bone; JN; 1998 Jun, 128:6, 1051-3
Bikle; Alcohol Induced Bone Disease; WRND; 1993; 73; 53-79
Boivin et al; Fluoride Helps Bone Density; WRND; 1993; 73; 80-103
Bonjour et al; Calcium Helps Prepubertal Girls; JCI; 1997; 99:1287; 1287-1294
Boyd Eaton et al; Calcium in Evolutionary Perspective; AJCN; 1991; 54; 281S-7S
Calvo et al; High Phosphorous, Low Calcium Diets Provoke Unfavorable PTH; JCEM; 1990 May; 70 (5):1334-40
Ekenman; Bone Density in Medieval Skeletons; CTI ; (1995); 56; 355-58
Ellis et al; Vegetarians Have Healthier Bones; AJCN; 25; June 1972; 555-8
Feskanich; Milk and Bone Fractures (Nurses Health Study); AJPH; 1997; 87; 992-997
Hegsted et al; Calcium Loss with Protein in Young Women; J Nutr; III; 244-51; 1981
Johnson, et al; Protein Intake on Urinary and Fecal Calcium in Adult Males; JN; 100; 1425-1430
Kalkwarf et al; Calcium Supplements Don't Help Lactating Women; NEJM; 1997; 337; 523-8
Karkkainen et al; Parathyroid Hormone Response to 4 Calcium Rich Foodstuffs; AJCN; 1997; 65; 1726-30
Kerstetter JE; et al; Protein-restricted Diet Increases PTH. AJCN; 1997 Nov, 66:5, 1188-96
Kerstetter; Protein Increases Urinary Calcium; J Nutr; 120;134-136; 1990
Licata; Monitoring Calcium Intake and Absorption; WRND; 1993; vol. 73; 27-52
Linkswiler et al; Protein Induced Hypercalciuria; Fed Proc; 1981; July 40:9, 2429-33
Lloyd et al; Caffeine Does Not Affect Bone Health in Older Women; AJCN; 1997; 65; 1826-30
Lutz; Protein Intake and Calcium Status and Acid-Base Status; AJCN; 1984; 39; 281-288
Mazes; Bone Content of North Alaskan Eskimos; AJCN; 27; 916-925; 1974
McClellan et al; Prolonged meat diets and metabolism of N, Ca and P; CC; XLVI; 1930; 669.
New et al; Fruit Best for Bone Health; AJCN; 1997; 65; 1831-9
Nilas; Calcium Intake and Osteoporosis; WRND; 1993 73; 1-26
Schuette; Protein Induced Hypercalciuria in Older People; JN, 1980 Feb, 110:2, 305-15
Simopoulos (ed.); Osteoporosis: Nutritional Aspects; WRND 1993: 73
Spencer et al; Osteoporosis, Ca Requirement; Ca Loss Factors; CGM; 1987 May; 3 (2):389-402
Trinidad et al; Calcium Absorption in the Colon; Nutrition; 1999; 15; 529-533
Watkins et al; Importance of Dietary Fats and Bone Building; WRND; 1997; vol. 82; 250-59
Wood; High Calcium Diets Reduce Zinc Balance; AJCN;1997;65;1803-9
Wyshak et al; Carbonated Beverages, Calcium, Ca/P Ratio and Bone Fractures; JAH; 1994 May; 15(3): 210-5
Yuen et al; Effect of Dietary Protein on Calcium metabolism in Man; NAR; 54; 447-459
Zarkadas; Sodium Chloride is Risk Factor for Osteoporosis; AJCN; 1989 Nov; 50 (5): 1088-94
Zemel; Dietary Protein Exerts a Significant Calciuretic Effect; AJCN 1988 Sep, 48:3 (S), 880-3

Cancer
AICR; Plant Based Diets Fight Cancer; AICR Guidelines; October 1997
Cummings; High Fruit and Vegetable and Low Meat Diets Combat Cancers; BMJ 1998;317:1636-1640
Djuric et al; Fruit and Vegetables Cut Breast Cancer Risk; JADA; 1998;98:524-528
Giovannucci ; Coffee May Cut Colon Cancer Risk; AJE; 1998;147:1043-1052.
Giovannucci; Selenium May Lower Prostate Cancer Risk; JNCI; 1998;90:1184-1185, 1219-1224.
Giovannucci; Tomatoes, Lycopene, Combat Cancer: Review of the Epidemiological Literature; JNCI; Feb. 17, 1999
Glaspy; Diet Fish Oil Reduce Breast Cancer Risk; JNCI; 1997; 89:1123-1131
Goodman; Plant Food, Soy and Fibre Diet Cuts Endometrial Cancer; AJE; (1997;146(4):294-306)
Gronbaek et al; Wine not Carcinogenic, Beer and Spirits are; BMJ 1998;317:844-848.

Hunter et al; DDT, PCB Exposure Not Linked To Breast Cancer; NEJM; 1997;337:1253-1258,1303-1304.
Jansen; Dietary Fibre Combats Colorectal Cancer; IJC 1999;81:174-179.
Katiyar; Tea Combats Cancer; WRND; 1996; vol. 79; 154-84
Knekt et al; Flavonoids and Antioxidants Combat Cancers; AJE; 1997; 146;223
Knekt; Selenium Deficiency is Risk for Lung Cancer; AJE; 1998;148:975-982
Kohlmeier; Fried Foods and Trans Fatty Acids Linked To Breast Cancer; CEPB; 1997; 6:705-710
Lagergren; Obesity is a Strong Risk Factor For Cancer of the Esophagus; AIM; 1999;130:883-890.
Leaf and Kang; n-3 Fatty Acids and Cardiovascular Disease; WRND; 1998; vol. 83; 24-37
Lee et al; Soy Compound has Anti Cancer Effect; JNCI; (1998;90:381-388)
Martinez; Link Between Obesity, Exercise and Colon Cancer Found; JNCI; 1999; **91:950-953.**
Michaud et al; Cruciferous Vegetables Combat Bladder Cancer in Men; JNCI; 1999; 91:605-613.
Nehlig; Coffee not Carcinogenic - review; WRND;1996; vol. 79; 185-221
Ruoslahti; How Cancer Spreads; SA; Sept 1996;42-47
Silverman et al; Obesity Raises Pancreatic Cancer Risk; JNCI; 1998;90:1710-1719.
Singh et al; White Meat Linked to Colon Cancer Risk; AJE; 1998;148:761-774.
Sutton; Phytochemicals Combat Cancer, SA; Sept 1996
Trichopoulos et al; Causes of Cancer; SA; Sept 1996; 50
Vines; Bananas Keep Cancer at Bay; NS; 25 June 1994
Zhang; Carotenoids and Dietary Vitamins Reduce Breast Cancer Risk; JNCI; 1999; 91:547-556.
Zino et al; Fruits and Vegetables Fight Cancer; BMJ; 1997;314:1787-1791

Cardiovascular Disease

Appel L J et al; 'DASH' Study - Dietary Effect on Blood Pressure; NEJM; 1997;336;1117-24
Ellis; Childhood Visceral Fat Predicts CVD; AJCN; 1997; 65; 1887-8
Enos et al; Coronary Disease in US Soldiers Killed in Korea; JAMA July 18 1953 vol. 152 no. 12
Kafatos et al; CHD and Dietary Changes in Crete:7 Countries Study Revisited; AJCN; 1997; 65; 1882-6
Khaw et al; Potassium and Stroke; NEJM; Jan 29 1987; 316; no.5; 235
Klatsky et al; Various Alcoholic Beverages and Risk for CAD; AJC; 1997; 80; 416-420
Lawn; SA; Lipoprotein(a) in Heart Disease; June 1992; 26-32
Leren; Oslo Diet Heart Study; Circulation; vol. XLII; Nov. 1970; 935-42
MacNamara; Coronary Artery Disease in US Combat Casualties in Vietnam; JAMA; May17; vol. 216; no7
Moore; Pathogenesis of Arteriosclerosis; Metabolism; vol. 34; no.12; Suppl. 1 (December); 1985;13-16
Mosca et al; Antioxidant Vitamins Reduce LDL Oxidation; JACC; 1997; 30; 392-9
Nutrition Reviews; Plant Foods Combat Atherosclerosis; NRW; June 1977vol. 35; no 6; 148-150
Osterud et al; Marine Oils Improve Cardiovascular Indicators; Lipids; 1995 Dec; 30(12):1111-8
Pearson et al; Thrombotic Hemostatic Factors and CVD; AJCN; 1997; 65 (s); 1674S-82S
Petroni et al; Olive Oil Phenols Inhibit Platelet Aggregation and AA Metabolism.; WRND; 1994; 75; 169-172
Pyoraia et al; Helsinki Policemen Study: Hyperinsulinemia Predicts CHD; Circulation; 1998; 98:398-404
Sirtori; Plant (Soybean) Protein Lowers Cholesterol; Lancet; Feb5; 1977
Sowers et al; Insulin and Hypertension; AJH; 1993; 6; 260S-270S
Stout; Overview of Insulin and Atherosclerosis; Metabolism; vol. 34; no. 12; suppl. 1; December; 1985; 7-12
Suckling; Atherosclerosis; in Encyclopedia of Human Biology; 1991; Academic Press, Inc.
Tobian et al; Salt Injures Arteries Without Necessarily Raising Blood Pressure; Hypertension; 1990; 15:900-903
Woo et al; Chinese less Susceptible than Whites to have Endothelial Dysfunction; JACC; 1997; 30; 113-8

Comparative Nutrition

Andrews et al; Evolutionary Model for Feeding Behavior; in Food Acquisition & Processing of Primates (P)
Blaxter; Comparative Nutrition; in Diet of Man: Needs and Wants (P)
Blaxter; Comparative Nutrition; Zoological Society of London; 198th meeting; March 15 1968
Chivers et al; Food, Form and Function; in The Digestive System of Mammals (P)
Coe; Niche Structure and Habitats; in Food acquisition & Processing of Primates (P)
Kortland; Habitat, Foraging and Diet in Chimpanzees; in Food Acquisition and Processing (P)
Ripley; Environmental Niches and Feeding Behavior, in Food acquisition & Processing of Primate (P)

Composition of Foods

McCance and Widdowson; The Composition of Foods [for Acid/Alkali Indices]; HMSO; 1960
McCance and Widdowson; The Composition of Foods; HMSO; 5th Edition
USDA; Composition of Foods: Raw, Processed, Prepared; Nutrient Database for Standard Reference, No. 12

Dietaries

Abdullah et al; Vegans - Nutrient Intake and Health Status; AJCN; 34; 2464-2477; 198
Chen & Xu; Chinese Dietary Patterns; WRND; 1996; vol. 79; 133-153
Darby et al; Food: The Gift of Osiris; Academic Press; 1977
Dwyer et al; Nutritional Status of Vegetarian Children; AJCN; 1982; 35; 204
Fidanza; Diets in Greece and Rome; PFNS; vol. 3, 79-99;1979
Gjonca; Albanian Paradox; Lancet; 1997; 350; 1815-17

Johanssen; Trace Element Status and Vegetarian Diet; AJCN; 1992;55:885-90
Keys; Seven Countries Study; Harvard U.P.; 1980
Labadarios; South African Eating Patterns; WRND; 1996; vol. 79; 70-108
Lee; Aboriginal Diet and Health; WRND; 1996; 79; 1-52
McCarrison; A Good Diet and a Bad One; IJMR; 1926; 14; 649-54
McCarrison; Effect of Deficient Dietaries on Monkeys; BMJ; Feb 21 1921; 249
McCarrison; Diseases Of Faulty Nutrition; Nutrition And Health; McCarrison Society; Faber And Faber; 1982
McCarrison; National Ill Health; Nutrition and Health; The McCarrison Society; Faber and Faber; 1982
McCarrison; Nutritive Values of Wheat, Paddy and Other Grains; IJMR; 1926:14;631-639
McCarrison; Problems of Food, Especially in India; JRSA; Jan 2 1925; 137-153
Milton; Nutritional Characteristics of Wild Primate Foods; Nutrition; 1999; vol. 15; 488-498
Naughton et al; Australian Aboriginal Meat is Very Low Fat, High in EFA's; Lipids; 1986; Nov; 21(11): 684-90
Nestle (Gen. Editor); Mediterranean Diets: Science and Policy Implications; AJCN; June 1995; vol. 61; no. 6(S)
O'Dea; Australian Aboriginal Traditional Diet Produces Good Vital Signs; MJA; 1988 Feb 15; 148(4); 177-80
O'Dea; Australian Aboriginal: Traditional Diet Characteristics; PTRSLBBS; 1991 Nov 29; 334 (1270); 233-40
Paoli; Rome: Its Life People and Customs; Chapter V - Food, Chapter VI - Banquets; Longmans; London; 1963
Reddy et al; Vegetarians: Essential Fatty Acids in Maternal Milk; WRND; 1994; vol. 75; 102- 104
Renaud, et al; Cretan Mediterranean Diet and Prevention of CHD; AJCN; June 1995; vol. 61; 6(S)
Renaud; Canola Oil Used for the Lyon Diet Heart Study; Personal Communication; July 22, 1997
Sanders et al; Vegans - Health Status and Fatty Acids; AJCN; 31:805-813;1978
Simopoulos et al; Purslane; WRND; 1995; vol. 77; 47-74
Sinclair; Diet of Canadian Indians and Eskimos; Symposium Proceedings; vol. 12; 69-82;1953
Willett; What We Should Eat; Science; vol. 264; 22 April.94

Digestive Tract

Auricchio; Gut Absorption: Racial differences; in Food, Nutrition and Evolution (P)
Caspary; Physiology and Intestinal Absorption; AJCN; 1992; Jan; 55 (1 Suppl.); 299S-308S
Corthier et al; Bacterial Toxins in G.I.; WRND
Cummings et al; Effects of Carbohydrates in the Gut; AJCN; 1995; 61(S); 938S
Edwards; Nutrition and Gut Microflora; PNS; 1993; 52; 375-82
Lin et al; Fibre Slows Intestinal Transit; AJCN; 1997; 65; 1840-4
Macfarlane; Fermentation in the Colon; PNS; 1993; 52; 367-373
Marteau et al; Fate of Transiting Micro-organisms in Gut; WRND 1993; vol 74; 1-21
Mathias et al; Hyperinsulinemia, EFA deficits Promote Endometriosis and Gut Dysfunction; FS; 1998 Jul; 70(1): 81-8
McCarrison; Deficiency Disease and Gastro-intestinal Disorder; BMJ; June 19 1920; 822
McCarrison; Rice and Intestinal Lesions; IJMR; 1919-1920; no VII; 7; 283 - 307
Milton; Primate Diets and Gut Morphology; in Food and Evolution (P)
Moreau; Intestine: Immune Response to Antigens; WRND; 1993; vol. 74; 22-57
O'Keefe et al; Milk Tolerance and the Malnourished African; EJCN; 1990 Jul; 44 (7): 499-504
Roland et al; Intestinal Flora and Xenobiotic Enzymes - Health Consequences; WRND; 1993; vol. 74; 123 - 148
Rothman; Regulation of Digestive Reactions by the Pancreas; in Handbook of Physiology (P)
Russell; Gut Changes with Age; AJCN; 1992; 55; 1203S-7S
Stone-Dorshow et al; Gas caused by Fructo-oligosaccharide; AJCN; 1987; 46; 61-5 ABS
Szylis; Effects of Carbohydrate Fermentation; WRND; 1993 vol. 74; 88-122
Truswell; Dietary Fibre and Health; WRND; 1993; vol. 72; 148-164
Vines; Junk Foods Grow Bad Bacteria; NS; Aug 8 1998

Energy Metabolism, Diabetes and Obesity

Bistrian; Protein Sparing Fast; JAMA; Nov 17; 1978; vol. 240; no. 21.
Brand-Miller; Evolutionary Aspects of Diet and Insulin Resistance; WRND; 1999; 84; 74-105
Crapo; Glucose, Insulin, Glucagon Responses to Complex Carbohydrates; AJCN; 34; 184-190;1981
Day et al; Insulin & Glucagon responses to Normal Meals; CE; 1978; 9; 443-454
Estrich et al; Hyperglycemia: Effect of Co-ingestion of Fat and Protein; Diabetes; vol. 16; no 4; 232
Fajans et al; Protein: Effect on Plasma Insulin; Diabetes; 18:523-528; Aug 1969
Flatt; Use and Storage of Carbohydrates and Fat; AJCN; 1995;61S:952S-9S
Floyd et al; Insulin Stimulated by Amino Acids; JCI; vol 45 no 9; 1966; 1487-01
Ford et al; Weight Change and Diabetes Incidence; AJE; 1997; 146; 214-22
H:son Nilsson; Glycogen after Glucose and Fructose; SJCLI; 33; 5-10; 1974
Hirsch; Carbohydrates: Key Issues for the Future; AJCN; 1995;61(S);996S
Jenkins et al; Low GI Foods in Hyperlipidemia; AJCN;1987;46;66-71(A)
Larner; Insulin and Glucagon; in Encyclopedia of Human Biology; vol. 4; 1991; API
Lienhard; How Cells Absorb Glucose; SA; Jan 1992.
Nevins; Sugars - Origins and Conversions; AJCN; 1995;61(S);915S-21S
Reiser et al; Fructose: Effect on Insulin During Post-prandial Hyperglycemia; AJCN; 1987; 45; 580-7

Rolls; Carbohydrates, Fats and Satiety; AJCN; 1995; 61(S);960
Simopoulos; Fatty Acids, Hyperinsulinemia and Obesity; FRBM; vol. 17; no 4; 367-72; 1994
Sirtori et al; Diabetes: Effect of n-3 Fatty Acids; AJCN; 1997; 65; 1874-81
Spiller et al; Protein and Sugar Dose: Effect on Glucose and Insulin; AJCN;1987; 46; 474-80
Thompson; Phytic Acid: Effect on Calcium and Blood Glucose; AJCN; 1987; 46; 467-73
UK Prospective Diabetes Study Group; Diabetes: Improved by BP Control; BMJ; vol. 317; 12 Sept 1998; 703
Zimmett et al; Diabetes in the South Pacific; Diabetes/Metabolism Reviews; vol. 6; no. 2; 91-124;1990

Evolutionary Anthropology
Brothwell; Diet Variation and Early Humans; Domestication of Plants and Animals
Foley; Hominids, Humans and Hunter-gatherers: An Evolutionary Perspective; in Hunters and Gatherers (P)
Garn; Stature and Evolution; in Food, Nutrition and Evolution (P)
Hassan; Size, Density and Growth Rate of Hunter-Gatherer Populations; in Population, Ecology, & Social Evolution (P)
Kappelman; Giants: Body Mass of Neanderthals; Nature;vol.387;8 May1997
Kay & Covert; Extinct Primate diets; in Food Acquisition & Processing of Primates (P)
Kretchmer; Food - a Selective Agent in Evolution; in Food Acquisition & Processing of Primates (P)
Milton; Primate Diets and Gut Morphology; in Food and Evolution (P)
Ruff; Climate and Body Shape; JHE; 1991; 21; 81-105
Stini; Body Composition and Nutrient Reserves in Evolutionary Perspective; in Food, Nutrition and Evolution (P)
Tattersall; Out of Africa, Again and Again; SA; April 1997
Wilson et al; Recent African Genesis of Humans; SA; April; 1992

Evolution of Food Supply
Frezal; Food and Genetic Selection; in Food Man & Society (P)
Hamilton III; Primate Diets and Human Over-consumption of Meat; in Food and Evolution (P)
Hawkes; How Much Food do Foragers Need?; in Food and Evolution (P)
Milton; Diet and Primate Evolution; SA; Aug 1993; 70-77
Molleson; Eloquent Bones of Abu Hureyra; SA; 1994 vol. 2; 71;2;70-75
Pellett; Problems in Assessment of Human Nutritional Status; in Food and Evolution: (P)
Simoons; Geography and Man's Food Quest; Food Man & Society (P)
Ucko & Dimbleby; Domestication of Plants and Animals (P)
White; Food & History; in Food, Man & Society (P)
Winterhalder; Analysis of Hunter Gatherer Diets; in: Food and Evolution (P)
Zohary, Hopf; Domestication of Plants in the Old World (P)

Evolutionary Health and Nutrition
Angel; Pleistocene Health; in Population, Ecology & Social Evolution (P)
Blumenschine; Carcass Consumption Sequences; JHE; 1986; 15; 639- 659
Boyd Eaton et al; Dietary Intake of Polyunsaturated Fatty Acids During the Paleolithic; WRND; 1998; 83 12-23
Boyd Eaton; Evolutionary Aspects of Diet; WRND;1997; vol. 81; 26-37
Boyd Eaton; Evolutionary Perspective of Human Nutrition; JN; 126;1732-1740;1996
Cordain; Cereal Grains: Humanity's Double-Edged Sword; WRND; 1999; 84; 19-73
Eaton; Paleolithic Nutrition; NEJM; 1985; 312; 5; 283
Harris; History of Human Subsistence; in Food Nutrition & Evolution (P)
Peters and O'Brien; Hominid Plant Foods in Sub-tropical Africa; in Digestive System in Mammals (P)
Phillipson; Paleonutrition and Modern Nutrition; WRND; 1997; vol. 81; 38-48
Sept; Plant Foods and Early Hominids; JHE; 1986; 15; 751-770
Simopoulos; Overview of Evolutionary Aspects of n-3 Fatty Acids in the Diet; WRND; 1998; vol. 83; 1-11
Speth; Early Hominid Hunting; JHE; 1989; 18;329-343
Wells; Prehistoric Diseases; in PFNS; vol. 1; no 11; 729-779; 1975
Yudkin; Archeology and the Nutritionist; in Domestication of Plants and Animals (P)

Exercise
Chen: Evolutionary Aspects of Exercise; WRND; 1999; 84; 106-117
Cordam et al; Exercise: Evolutionary Aspects; WRND; 1997; 81; 49-60
Coyle; Substrate Utilization During Exercise; AJCN; 1995; 61S:968S-79S
Guidelines on Exercise for Older Adults; MSSE; 1998;30:992-1008.
Henson et al; Exercise: Effect on Resting Energy Expenditure; AJCN; 1987; 46; 893-9
Horton; Exercise and Insulin; DMR; vol. 2; nos. 1&2; 1986
Simopoulos and Pavlou (eds); Nutrition and Fitness for Athletes; WRND; 1992; vol. 71
Simopoulos; Nutrients, Physical Activity and Genes Expression; WRND; 1997; 81; 61-71
Stallings; Nutritional Needs of the Exercising Child; WRND; 1997; 81; 90-97 American College of Sports Medicine;
U.S. Surgeon General; The Influence of Regular Physical Activity on Health; .July 1996

Foodstuffs and Technology
Alexander & Coursey; Yams; in; Domestication of Plants and Animals; Ucko & Dimbleby; Duckworth;1969
Chinachoti; Carbohydrates and Sweeteners; Functionality in Foods; AJCN; 1995;61(S); 922S

Coca-Cola; Coca Cola Products: Ingredients; May 1998
Ellwood; Sugar Alcohols - Energy Content; AJCN; 1995; 62(Suppl);1169S-74S
FDA; Caffeine Content of Different Products; US Food and Drug Administration
Flack; Emulsifying Agents in Modern Food Production (especially bread); FSTT; 1; (4)
Goldenfields; Rapeseed Oil (Goldenfields): Fatty Acid Profile; Personal Communication; June 1998
Hanover; Fructose: Manufacture, Composition and Applications; AJCN 1993; 58(S); 724S-32S
Levin; Sugar Substitutes - Characteristics and Benefits; AJCN; 1995; 62(Suppl); 1161S-8S
Spectrum Naturals; Canola Oil (Spectrum Naturals): Fatty Acid Profiles; Customer Information; June 1999
Spectrum Naturals; Canola Spread (Spectrum Naturals): Fatty Acid Profiles; Customer Information; June 1999
Spectrum Naturals; Flax Oils (Spectrum Naturals): Fatty Acid Profiles; Customer Information; June 1999
Stegink; Aspartame: A Model for Clinical Testing; AJCN; 1987; 46; 204-15
Wesson; Canola Oil (Wesson): Fatty Acid Profile; Personal Communication; June 1999

Food Toxicity

Hladik; Alcaloides de la Foret Dense; La Terre et La Vie; Tome XXXI; no 4 Oct-Dec; 1977
Levine Pesticides in Humans; in Handbook of Pesticide Toxicology; vol. 1, General Principles, 1991, API
PSD; Acceptable Daily Intakes; Pesticide Safety Directorate (UK); Personal Communication; 18 June 1997
Waterman; Feeding and Plant Chemistry: in Food Acquisition and Processing (P)

Glycemic, Insulin and Satiety Indexes

Bornet et al G.I. and I.I. of Six Starches, Alone and in Mixed Meals;; AJCN;1987;45;45-588-95
Brand-Miller et al; G.I. of Sugary Foods: Natural vs. Added Sugar; BJN; 1995; 73; 613-623
Brand-Miller; G.I. of Rices; AJCN; 1992; 56; 1034-6
Bucalossi et al; G.I.. and I.I. of Different Carbohydrates (ice cream); DNM; 3; 143-151; 1990
Bukar; G I of Frozen Desserts; DC; 13:382-85;1990
Foster-Powel et al; G.I. Glycemic Indices: International Tables; AJCN 1995, 62, 871S-93S
Gannon et al; Insulin and Glucose Response to Milk and Fruit; Diabetologia;1986;29;784-791
Granfeldt; G I of Pasta Varieties and Pasta Bread; EJCN; (1991); 45; 489-99
Heaton; Particle Size: Effect on G.I. and I. I. .of Wheat, Maize, Oats; AJCN;1988;47;675-82
Hermansen et al; G.I. of Banana Ripeness; Diabetic Medicine; 1992; 9; 739 - 743
Holt et al; An Insulin Index of Foods; AJCN; 1997; 66:1264-76
Holt et al; Satiety: An Index of Common Foods; EJCN; 1995; 49; 675-90
Holt; Glucose, Insulin and Satiety Responses; EJCN; 1996; 50; 788-97
Jenkins et al; G.I. Effects of Starch/Protein Interaction; AJCN; 1987; 45; 946-51
Jenkins et al; G.I. of Legumes; Diabetologia; 1983; 24; 257-264
Jenkins et al; G.I. of Traditional Wheat and Rye Bulgar and Pumpernickel Bread; AJCN;43;april 1986; 516-20
Jenkins et al; G.I. Wholemeal Compared to Whole-grain; BMJ; 297; 15 Oct 1988
Jenkins et al; Glycemic Index of Foods; AJCN; 34 362-366; 1981
Mani et al; G.I. of Conventional Indian Carbohydrate Meals; BJN;1992;68;445-450
Monge et al; G.I. and Insulin Index (I.I.) of Two Types of Spaghetti; DNM; 3; 239-246; 1990
Vorster et al; G I of Butter Beans plus Sugars; AJCN; 1987; 45; 575-9
Westphal et al; G I Related to Mixed Glucose and Protein; AJCN; 1990:52:267-72
Wolever et al; G.I. of 102 foods; NR; vol. 14; no 5; 651- 669; 1994
Wolever et al; G.I. of Fruits and Product in Diabetics; IJFSN; 1993;43;205-212
Wolever et al; G.I. of Regular and Parboiled Rice; NR; vol. 6; 349-357;1986
Wolever; G.I. and Insulin Index of Mixed Meals; JN; 126; 2807-12; 1996
Wolever; G.I. of Pasta: Effect of Surface Area, Cooking and Protein Enrichment; Diabetes Care; 1986; 9; 401-404

Immune System; Auto-immune diseases, allergies etc

Buisseret; Cow's Milk Allergy in Children; Lancet; Feb 11, 1978.
Calder; n-3 Fatty Acids and Immune Function; AER; 1997; 37: 197-237
Chandra and Chandra; Nutrition, Immune Response and Outcome; PFNS; 1986; 0(1-2):1-65
Clark et al; n-3 fatty acid in Systemic Lupus Erythematosus; KI; 1989 Oct; 36 (4):653-60
Comstock; Antioxidants, Rheumatoid Arthritis and Lupus; Annals of Rheumatic Diseases;1997;56;323-325
Coppo et al; Gluten-Free Diet Relieves Mucosal Immune System; CN; 1986; Aug; 26(2):72-82
Corman; Relationship Between Nutrition, Infection and Immunity; MCNA; 1985 May; 69(3):519-31
Endres; n-3 Fatty Acids and Human Cytokine Synthesis; Lipids; 1996 Mar; 31 Suppl: S239-42
Fernandes; Dietary Lipids and Autoimmune Disease; CII; 1994 Aug; 72(2):193-7
Garritson et al; Effect of Major Dietary Modifications on Immune System; CP; 1995 Jul-Aug; 3(4): 239-46
Gibney et al; Effects on the Immune System of n-3 Fatty Acids; EJCN; 1993 Apr; 47(4):255-9
Gogos et al; Immunodeficiency Restored by n-3 Fatty Acids and Vitamin E; Cancer; 1998 Jan 15; 82(2):395-402
Hannigan; Diet and Immune Function; BJMS; 1994 Sep; 51(3): 252-9
Holman; Importance of n-3 Fatty Acids in Human Health; JN 1998 Feb; 128(Suppl):427S-433S
Hughes; Beta-Carotene: Effect on Immune Function of Non-Smokers; JLCM; 1997 Mar; 129(3): 309-17
Imoberdorf; Designer Diets in Cancer; SCC; 1997 Sept; 5(5):381-6

Kelley et al; Low Copper Diet Depresses Immune Function; AJCN; 1995 Aug 62(2): 412-6
Kelley et al; Low Fat Diet Improves Immune System Indices; CII; 1992 Feb; 62(2): 240-4
Kremer et al; Rheumatoid Arthritis Improved by High-Dose Fish Oil; AR; 1995; Aug; 38 (8): 1107-14
Lichtenstein; Allergy and Immune System; SA; sept 1993 85-83
Mainous et al; Nutrition and Infection; SCNA; 1994; June; 74(3):659-76
Mendez et al; Immune Enhancing Diet: Effects in Critically Injured Patients; JT; 1997 May; 42(5):933-40
Metzler et al; Role of Autoimmunity in Atherogenesis; WKW; 1998 May 22; 110(10):350-5
Meydani; Killer Cell Cytoxicity Mediated by Fish Oil and Tocopherol; JN 1988 Oct; 118(10): 1245-52
Nossal; The Immune System; SA; Sept 1993 21-30
Reffett; Dietary Selenium and Vitamin E: Effect on Immune Response; JAS 1988 Jun; 66(6): 1520-8
Sandstrom et al; Acrodermatitis and Zn, Cu Metabolism and Immune Function; APAM; 1994 Sep; 148(9): 980-5
Schreiner et al; Diet and Kidney Disease; PSEBM; 1991 May; 197(1):1-11
Soyland et al; Very Long Chain Fatty Acids on Immune Related Skin Disease; EJCN; 1993 Jun; 47(6):381-8
Steinman; Autoimmune Disease; SA; Sept 1993 75-83
Wan et al; Nutrition, Immune Function and Inflammation: an Overview; PNS; 1989 Sep; 48(3):315-35 Weber;
Williams et al; Stress, Immune System; and n-6 fatty acids; PLFA; 1992 Oct; 47(2):165-70
Vitamin E and Human Health: Immune Response etc; Nutrition; 1997 May 13(5):450-60

Lipids

Baba et al; Effects of Canola Oil and Olive Oils on Plasma Lipids; NR; 1999; vol. 19; 601-612
Bracco; Triglyceride Structure: Effect on Fat Absorption; AJCN 1994;60S:1002S-9S
Budowski & Crawford; n-3 and Regulation of Arachidonic Acid, n-6/n-3 ratio; PNS; 1985; 44; 221-29
Caggiula et al; Dietary Fat and CHD risk; AJCN; 1997; 65(S); 1597S-610S
Crawford; Fatty Acid Ratios in Free-living and Domestic animals; Lancet; June 22; 1968; 1329-33
Denke; Beef and Beef Tallow - Stearic Acid; AJCN;1994;60S;1044S-9S
Denke; Cocoa Butter and Serum Lipids: History; AJCN; 1994; 60S; 1014S-6S
Dietschy; LDL & HDL Regulation; AJCN; 1995; 65 (S) 1581S
Dietschy; LDL and HDL Regulation: Theory; AJCN; 1997; 65S;1581S-9S
Emken; Stearic Acid: Metabolism Relative to other Fatty Acids; AJCN; 1994; 60S; 1023S-8S
Frankel et al; Red Wine Inhibits LDL Oxidation; Lancet; vol. 341; Feb. 20; 1993
Grundy; Stearic Acid Compared to the Effect of Other Fatty Acids on Cholesterol; AJCN; 1994; 60S; 986S-90S
Harris; n-3 Fatty Acids and Lipoproteins in Humans; AJCN 65(S); 1645S-54S
Hellerstein et al; Lipogenesis of Fat in Liver; JCI; 1991; 87; 1841-52
Hornstra et al; Fatty Acid Profile and Vitamin E: Effect on LDL Peroxidation; WRND;1994;75;149-154
Houwelingen et al; Fish: Effect on Cardiovascular Indices; AJCN; 1987; 46; 424-36
Howell et al; Blood Lipid Responses to Diet; AJCN; 1997; 65; 1747-64
Insull et al; Fatty Acid: Comparison Between Japanese and Americans; JCI; vol.48; 1969; 1313
Kagawa; Eicosapolynoic Acid Levels of Japanese Islanders; JNSV; 28; 441-53; 1982
Katan; Oils, Lipoproteins and CHD; AJCN; 1995; 61(S); 1368S-73S
Kisella; PUFA's and Eicosanoid Synthesis; 1990; JNB; 1; March; 123
Kris-Etherton et al; Chocolate Feeding: Stearic Acid; AJCN; 1994; 60(S); 1029S-36S
Kris-Etherton; Plasma Lipids and Lipoproteins; AJCN; 1997; 65(S); 1628S-44S
Kritchevsky; Stearic Acid Metabolism and Atherogenesis; AJCN:1994:60S:997S-1001S
Kummerow; Eggs and Serum Cholesterol; AJCN; 30; 664-73; 1977
Lien; EFA Ratio in Infant Formulas; WRND; 1994; vol. 75; 92-95
Lossonczy et al; Fish: Effect on Serum Lipids; AJCN; 31; 1340-46; 1978
Mensinck; Trans-Fatty acids: Alternatives; WRND; 1994; 75; 190
Miraglio; Energy Values of Fat Substitutes; AJCN;1995; 62(suppl); 1175S-9S
N Salem et al; n-3 Fatty Acids: are they Essential?; WRND;1993;72; 128-147
Nenseter et al; LDL's in Relation to Fatty acids and Anti-oxidants; WRND; 1994; vol 75; 144- 48
Nestel; Trans-fatty Acids on Lipoprotein levels; WRND; 1994; vol 75; 187-89
Richter et al; Lipoproteins and Vegetarians; NR; 1999; vol. 19; 545-554
Salem; Lipid Nutrition and Early Development; WRND; 1994; 75; 46-51
Scarborough; FDA Perspectives on Fats; AJCN 1997; 65(S); 1578S-80S
Siebert et al; Red Meat Compared with n-3 EFA's: Effects on cardiac arrhythmia; NR; 13; 1407-18; 1993
Simon et al; Fatty Acids and the Risk of Stroke; Stroke; 1995; 26; 778-782
Simopoulos; Fatty Acids, Obesity and Insulin Resistance; FRBM; vol. 17; no 4; 367-72; 1994
Sirtori et al; n-3 Fatty Acids and Diabetic Risk; AJCN; 1997; 65; 1874-81
Sugano et al; Trans-fatty Acids: Effect on Eicosanoid Production; WRND; 1994; 75; 179-182
Tzagournis; Triglycerides in Clinical Medicine; AJCN; 31; 1437-52; 1978
Vorster et al; High Egg, Low Fat Diets: Effect on Blood Lipids; AJCN; 1987;46;52-7
Wahle et al; Trans-fatty acids: Effect on Platelet Function; WRND; 1994; vol. 75; 183-86
Woollett et al; Long Chain Fatty Acids: Effect on LDL Metabolism; AJCN; 1994;60(S);991S

Zino; Fruit and Vegetables: Effect on Blood lipids and Anti-oxidants; BMJ; vol. 314; 21 June 1997

Longevity

Frolkis and Muradian; Dietary Factors for Life Span Prolongation; in Life Span Prolongation (P)
Huijbregts; Three Country Elderly Mortality and Diet Study; BMJ; 315; 5 July 1997
Kinsella; Changes in Life Expectancy; AJCN; 1992; 55; 1196S-1202S
Leaf: Gerontology; Hunza, Georgians, Vincambamba; Nutrition Today; Sept/Oct 1973
Trichopoulou et al; Diet and Overall Survival in Elderly People; BMJ; 311; 2 Dec 1995
Weindruch; Caloric Restriction and Aging; SA; Jan 1996; p. 32
WHO; Deaths Classed by Disease; World Health Statistics Annual; WHO 1995
WHO; Life Expectancy by Region; World Health Statistics Annual; WHO 1995

Macro- and Micro-nutrients

Aaseth; Selenium: Optimum Levels in Animal Products; NJAS; 1993; Suppl. 11; 121-126
Anon; Glucose Induced Chromium Excretion; AJCN; 31; July 1978; 1158-1161
Barclay; Selenium Content of UK foods; JFCA; 8; 307-318; 1995
Bogden et al; Zinc and Elderly Immune Response; AJCN; 1987; 46; 101-9; ABS
Crozier; Infant Antioxidants; WRND; 1994; 75; p. 96
Huis Int Veld; Probiotics - Health Aspects; FSTT; 12 (1) 1998
Ishikawa et al; Tea Flavonoids Suppress LDL Oxidation; AJCN; 1997; 66; 261-6
Levander; Rationale for the 1989 RDA for Selenium; JADA; 1991; 91; 1572-1576
Levine et al; Ascorbic Acid Requirements; WRND; 1993; 72; 114-127(A)
Mannan et al; Selenium in Diet Relates to Selenium in Breast Milk; AJCN; 1987; 46; 95-100
Miller & Mitchell; Protein: Optimization of Human Requirements ch. 4; Bureau of Foods, FDA, Washington DC.
Murphy et al; Vitamin E Intakes and Sources; AJCN; 1990; 52; 361
Paterson; Aspirin in Fruit; JCP; 1998; 51; 502-505
Payne; Safe Protein/Calorie Ratios in Children ; AJCN; 28; 281-86; 1975
Peterson et al; Flavonoids: Dietary Occurrence and Biochemical Activity; NR; 1998; 18; No 12; 1995-2018
Pizziol et al; Effects of Caffeine on Glucose Tolerance; EJCN; 1998 Nov; 52(11): 846-9
Poehlman et al; Effect of Caffeine and Exercise on Metabolism and Hormones; CJPP; 1989 Jan; 67(1):10-16
Prystai et al; Effect of Tea on Absorption of Ca, Cu, Fe Mg and Zn; NR; 1999; vol. 19; 167-177
Reddy et al; Calcium: Effect on Iron Absorption; AJCN; 1997; 65; 1820-5
Urbano et al; Bio-availability of Ca and P in Lentils; NR; 1999; vol. 19; 49-64
Yang et al; Selenium Intoxication in China; AJCN; 37; May 1983; 872-81
Ylaranta; Selenium Fertilization in Finland; NJAS; 1993; Suppl. No 11; 141-49

Metabolism

Aebi; Protein Metabolism and Amino Acid Balances; in Food Man & Society (P)
Floyd; Insulin Response to Protein; JCI; vol. 45; no 9; 1966
Jackson; Protein Metabolism in Chronic Malnutrition; PNS; 1993; 52; 1.10
McClelland; Prolonged Meat Diet - Kidneys and Ketosis; CC; XLV; 1930
Rennie et al; Protein: Effects of Malnutrition, Injury and Disease on Protein Metabolism; Lancet; Feb. 11 1984, 323
Suter; How Alcohol Puts on Fat; NEJM; 1992; 326; 983-7
Swanson et al; Fructose: Effects on Metabolism; AJCN; 1992; 55; 852-6
Westphal; Response to Glucose/Protein Doses; AJCN; 1990; 52; 267-72

Morphology

Boyde & Martin; Primate Enamel Microstructure; in Food Acquisition & Processing of Primates (P)
Chivers and Hladik; Gut Morphology and Diet in Mammals; JM; 166:337-386; 1980
Chivers and Langer; Gut Form and Function, in: The Digestive System of Mammals (P)
Chivers et al; Food Acquisition and Processing in Primates; in The Digestive System of Mammals (P)
Hiiemae; Functional Morphology of Jaw; in Food acquisition & Processing of Primates (P)
Hladik et al; Foods and Digestive System; in The Digestive System of Mammals (P)
Lalueza et al; Dietary Inferences through Buccal Microwear of Pleistocene Humans; AJPA; 1996; Jul; 100(3): 367-87
Langer: Weaning and Bypass Structures in Mammals; in The Digestive System of Mammals (P)
Langer; Comparison of Gastro-Intestinal Tract ratios; in The Digestive System of Mammals (P)
Lucas & Luke; Principles of Food Breakdown; in Food Acquisition and Processing of Primates (P)
Lucas; Categorization of Food Items Relevant to Oral Processing in: The Digestive System of Mammals (P)
Maier; Tooth Morphology and Diet; in Food Acquisition & Processing of Primates (P)
Milton; Primate Diets and Gut Morphology; Food and Evolution (P)
Moir; The Carnivorous Carnivore [Infant digestion]; in The Digestive System of Mammals (P)
Waterman; Feeding And Plant Chemistry; in Food Acquisition & Processing of Primates (P)

Phylogeny

Caccone et al; DNA Divergence in Hominoids; IJOE; Aug 1989; vol. 43; no 5; p925
Goodman et al; Primate Evolution at DNA Level; JME; (1990) 30: 260-266
Rogers; Phylogeny of Hominoids; JHE; 1993; 25; 201-215

Sibley et al; DNA Hybridization Evidence of Hominoid Phylogeny; JME (1990) 30;202-236 (A)

Tribal, Genetic and Regional Studies

Balke; Tarahumara Endurance Runners; AJPA; 23; 293-302; 1965
Ball; Pitcairn: The World's Oldest Commune; Nutrition Today; Sept/Oct; 1973
Booyens et al; Eskimo Diet: Benefits of Natural Cis and Absence of Trans PUFA; MH; 1986 Dec; 21(4): 387-408
Castro; Behavior Genetics of Food Intake; Nutrition; 1999; 15; 550-554
Connor; Tarahumara Indians of Mexico: Diet and Plasma Lipids; AJCN;31;1131-42;1978
Diabetologia; Amerindian Tribes: Glucose Tolerance; 1982; 23; 90-93
Feskens et al; Eskimos: Epidemiology and Fish Intake; ANYAS; 1993 Jun 14; 683: 9-15
Goran et al; Visceral Fat in White and Black Children; AJCN; 1997; 65; 1703-8
Groom; Tarahuramas Hearts; AHJ; March 1971; 81; 3; 304-14
Innis et al; Inuit Breast Milk: n-3 Fatty Acid Content; EHM; 1988 Dec; 18(2-3):185-9
Joffe; Kalahari Bushmen: Glucose Tolerance; BMJ; 23 Oct 1971; 206-8
Keenleyside; Pre-contact Alaskan Eskimos and Aleuts: Skeletal Evidence of Health; AJPA; 1998 Sep; 107(1):51-70
Leonard et al; Torres Strait Islanders: Modern Foods are Provoking Diabetes; ANJPH; 1995; Dec; 19(6): 589-95
Mann et al; Alaskan Eskimos: Health and Nutrition; AJCN; vol. 11, July 1962; 31-77
Merimee; African Pygmy: Metabolic Studies; JCI; 1972; vol. 51; 395-401
Neel; Yanomama: Health and Disease; Physician to the Gene Pool, Wiley 1994
O'Dea; Australian Aborigine: Glucose Tolerance Normalized by Traditional Diet; Diabetes; 33; June 1984; 596-603
Simoons; Geography of Celiac Disease; in Food, Nutrition & Evolution (P)
Simopoulos; Genetic Variation and Nutrition; WRND; 1999; vol. 84; 118-140
Truswell; Bushmen: Serum lipids Lancet; Sept 21 1968; 684
Wolever et al; Native Americans: Low Fibre, High Meat Diet Promotes Diabetes; AJCN; 1997; Dec; 66(6): 1470-4
Zimmet; Pacific Islanders: Non Insulin Dependent Diabetes; Diabetes; vol. 6; no. 2; 91-124; 1990

Journal Abbreviations: Concordance

AER	Advances in Enzyme Regulation
AICR	American Institute for Cancer Research
AIM	Annals of Internal Medicine
AJC	American J. of Cardiology
AJCN	American J. of Clinical Nutrition
AJE	American J. of Epidemiology
AHJ	American Heart J.
AJH	American J. of Hypertension
AJPA	American J. of Physical Anthropology
AJPH	American J. of Public Health
ANJPH	Australian J. of Public Health
ANYAS	Annals New York Academy of Sciences
APAM	Archives Pediatrics and Adolescent Medicine
AR	Arthritis Rheumatism
BJMS	British J. of Biomedical Science
BJN	British J. of Nutrition
BMJ	British Medical J.
CC	Clinical Calorimetry
CE	Clinical Endocrinology
CEBP	Cancer Epidemiology, Biomarkers and Prevention
CGM	Clin. Geriatr. Med.
CII	Clinical Immunology. Immunopathology
CJPP	Canadian J. of Physiology and Pharmacology
CN	Clinical Nephrology
CP	Cancer Practice
CTI	Calcified. Tissue International
DC	Diabetes Care
DNM	Diabetes Nutrition and Metabolism
EHD	Early Human Development
EJCN	European J. of Clinical Nutrition
FRBM	Free Radical Biology & Medicine
FS	Fertil Steril
FSTT	Food Science and Technology Today
IJC	International J. of Cancer
IJFSN	International J. of Food Sciences and Nutrition
IJMR	Indian J. of Medical Research
IJOE	Internatioal J. of Organic Evolution
JN	J. of Nutrition
JACC	J. of the American College of Cardiology
JADA	J. of the American Dietetic Association
JAH	J. of Adolescent Health
JAS	J. of Animal Science
JCEM	J. Clinical Endocrinology and Metabolism
JCI	J. of Clinical Investigation
JCP	J. of Clinical Pathology
JFCA	J. of Food Composition and Analysis
JHE	J. of Human Evolution
JLCM	J. Laboratory and Clinical Medicine
JM	J. of Morphology
JME	J. of Molecular Evolution
JNB	J. of Nutritional Biochemistry
JNCI	J. of the National Cancer Institute
JNSV	J. of Nutritional Science and Vitaminology
JRSA	J. of the Royal Society of Arts
JT	J. Trauma
KI	Kidney International
MCNA	Med. Clin. North Am.
MH	Medical Hypotheses
MJA	Medical J. of Australia
MSSE	Medicine and Science in Sports and Exercise
NAR	Nutritional Abstract Reviews
NJAS	Norwegian J. of Agricultural Sciences
NR	Nutrition Research
NRW	Nutrition Review
NS	New Scientist
PFNS	Progress in Food and Nutritional Science
PLFA	Prostaglandins, Leukotrienes and Essential Fatty Acids
PNS	Proceedings of the Nutrition Society
PSEBM	Proc. Soc. Exp. Biol. Med
PTRSLBS	Phil Trans Royal Society of London Biological Sciences
SA	Scientific American
SCC	Support-Care-Cancer
SCNA	Surg. Clin. North Am.
SJCLI	Scandinavian J. of Clinical Laboratory Investigation
WKW	Wien Klin. Wochenschr.
WRND	World Review of Nutrition and Dietetics

Publishers

API	Academic Press Inc
DW	Duckworth
HMSO	Her Majesty's Stationery Office
PP	Plenum Press
RP	Rodale Press
TUP	Temple University Press
UOC	University of Cambridge

Publications

Diet of Man: Needs and Wants; Symposium, Bath, UK; 17-22 April 1977; ed. Yudkin; 1978

Digestive System of Mammals; D J Chivers, P Langer; Press Syndicate; University of Cambridge; 1994

Domestication of Plants and Animals; Ucko & Dimbleby; Duckworth;1969

Domestication of Plants in the Old World; Zohary; Clarendon Press;Oxford;1993

Food Acquisition & Processing of Primates; Chivers, Wood and Bilsborough; New York, PP, 1984

Food and Evolution: Harris and Ross; 1987; TUP

Food, Man & Society; Walcher; I.O.S.H.D;1976; Plenum Press; NY; 1976

Food, Nutrition and Evolution; Walcher & Kretchmer; Masson; 1981

Handbook of Physiology; Rauner, Forte, Schultz, (eds.); Am Phys Soc.; Bethesda, Maryland 1989

Hunters and Gatherers; History, Evolution and Social Change; ed Ingold, Riches and Woodburn; Berg; Oxford; 1988

Life Span Prolongation; Frolkis and Muradian; CRC Press; Boca Raton, Florida; 1991

Population, Ecology, & Social Evolution.; Polgar; Mouton; 1975

Glossary

Acid	See **pH**
Alkali	See **pH**
Allergen	Any substance that triggers a state of allergy.
Amino Acid	Building blocks of **proteins.** There are about 20 of them that the body combines, in endless permutations, into the tens of thousands of proteins that the body needs. The body can make the vast majority of the huge number of the amino acids that it needs. Ten amino acids however are "essential" and have to be obtained from what we eat.
Aneurysm	A dilation in the wall of a blood vessel to form a blood-filled sac which can rupture and cause fatal hemorrhage.
Antioxidant	A chemical compound that neutralizes **free radicals** and the damage they cause. There are many antioxidants in plant food but rarely in animal products. Autoxidation proceeds by a chain reaction which continues as long as the chain carriers (**free radicals**) persist. Antioxidants, by reacting with chain carriers, terminate the oxidative chain reaction. There are a great number of food antioxidants of which the most common are vitamin C, vitamin E, zinc and selenium.
Atherosclerosis	A type of thickening and hardening of the medium- and large-sized arteries. It accounts for a large proportion of heart attacks **ischemic heart disease**, strokes and most **aneurysms** of the aorta.
Bad Carbohydrate	A **carbohydrate** that has a high **glycemic index**. It is capable of placing an unnatural stress on the body's blood sugar control mechanism. In this work Bad Carbohydrates are defined as having a **G.I.** higher than 65. See Chapter Five.
Base, Basic	See **pH.**
Bioflavonoid	A class of **micronutrients** that occur in plants. They cannot be made in the body but the body has need of most if not all of them. They therefore have to be obtained through eating plant food. There are six sub-classes of bioflavonoid: flavones, flavanones, flavonols, isoflavonoids, anthocyanins and flavans.
BMI	See **Body Mass Index.**
Body Mass Index	A useful measure of leanness or obesity. It is calculated as the individual's weight (in kg) divided by height (in meters) squared.
Borderline Carbohydrate	A **carbohydrate** that has a borderline **glycemic index**. It is *potentially* capable of placing an unnatural stress on the body's blood sugar control mechanism. In this work Borderline Carbohydrates are defined as having a **G.I.** between 35 and 65. See **Chapter Five.**
Calcium	A metallic element that is found compounded with other elements throughout nature, for example as chalk and limestone. In combination with phosphorous (calcium phosphate) it forms the major constituent of bones. Calcium is found in most plant foods and some animal products. It has the chemical symbol "Ca".
Candidiasis	An infectious disease produced by yeast-like funguses that are commonly found in the mouth, vagina, and intestinal tract. It is usually kept under control by the immune system and helpful bacteria. See **Chapter Eight.**
Carbohydrate	A multitude of compounds composed of carbon, oxygen and hydrogen. They form sugars, starches and plant cell walls. Carbohydrates are only found in plants. When they are digested they are ultimately converted into blood sugar (glucose). The human body is best designed for "slow" (low **G.I.**) carbohydrates as found in salads, vegetables and most fruits. It is also well adapted to **fructose**, the special sugar found in fruit. The human body is not well adapted to "fast" (high G.I.) carbohydrates. These are starches as found in cereals and potatoes, or sugars as found in table sugar and honey. See **Chapter Five**

Carnivore   Strictly speaking a member of the mammalian order Carnivore, literally "meat eaters". They are predators and comprise ten families. Examples from each family are dogs and foxes; bears and badgers; mongooses; hyenas; cats; sea lions; earless seals; and the walrus. Humans and other primates are not carnivores.

Cecum   The part of the gut that comes immediately after the small intestine and is the beginning of the colon (large intestine). Partially digested food passes to the cecum via a valve the (ileocecal valve). See **Chapter Four**.

Dairy products   Comprise milk (whole, skimmed, dried and condensed) and processed milk such as cream, yogurt (whole and skimmed) butter, cheeses and ice cream. The term applies to milk from all sources: cows (by far the most common), buffalo, goats, reindeer and sheep. Eggs are not a dairy product.

Diabetes   A disorder of **carbohydrate** metabolism resulting from insufficient production of, or reduced sensitivity to, insulin. See **Chapters Five** and **Eight**.

Diverticulitis   Condition in **diverticulosis** where the diverticula become infected and inflamed.

Diverticulosis   Diverticulosis is a condition where abnormal grape-like pockets ("diverticula") form in the wall of the intestine. It is a condition common in the West where a low fibre diet is common. There are usually no symptoms, although occasionally there may be bleeding.

DNA   Deoxyribonucleic Acid. This is the famous genetic code discovered by Watson and Crick and for which they were awarded a Nobel prize. DNA is present in every single body cell and is the blueprint from which the body is constructed and maintained. When new cells are born, or have to be maintained or change their function, the blueprint is consulted by other chemical compounds to define how the construction work should be carried out.

Eicosapentanoic Acid (E.P.A.)   A fatty acid commonly found in certain types of fish. In the body, the essential fatty acid, alpha-linolenic acid is converted into E.P.A. on its way to the production of "favorable" prostaglandins and similar substances. By consuming E.P.A. directly a short cut is taken to the formation of these helpful compounds.

Eicosonoid   Active compounds derived from **essential fatty acids**. There are three main classes: prostaglandins, thromboxanes and leukotrienes. These collectively are responsible for an amazing collection of body responses. They dilate or constrict blood vessels; excrete or retain urine; conserve or excrete sodium; modulate ovulation; stimulate uterine muscle contraction; provoke or calm menstrual cramps; induce therapeutic miscarriage; prevent or promote clotting; cause platelets to adhere to artery walls (**atherosclerosis**); enhance or inhibit inflammation; provoke or calm hypersensitivity (anaphylactic) reactions, allergies, and autoimmune diseases; modulate the functioning of the digestive tract; enhance or inhibit the contraction of the smooth intestinal muscles; inhibit stomach secretions; promote bone demineralization (resorption) and hypercalcemia (excess calcium in the blood).

Enzyme   A substance that speeds up a chemical reaction without itself being altered in the process. They are also known as catalysts. Enzymes intervene in a multitude of body reactions. An example is ptyalin in saliva. It converts starch to glucose in seconds when otherwise it would take hours.

Essential Fatty Acid   Of the twenty or more fatty acids only two are "essential", that is, they can only be obtained the diet. They are linoleic acid and alpha-linolenic acid. Informally they have been called vitamin F_1 and F_2 respectively. The recommended daily intake has not been formally determined, but it is commonly thought to be no more than about 1 gram each in an ideal ratio of 1:1. See **Chapter Five**.

Fats and Oils   Oils are simply fats that are liquid at room temperature. Anyone who has put a bottle of olive oil in the refrigerator will have seen how the oil turns solid – it becomes a fat. It is nevertheless exactly the same compound and readily turns back into oil at room temperature. Technically the words "fats" and "oils" are interchangeable. See **Chapter Five**.

Favorable Carbohydrate   A carbohydrate that has a low **glycemic index**. It is one that does not place an unnatural stress on the blood sugar control mechanism. In this work Favorable Carbohydrates are defined as having a **G.I.** below 35. See **Chapter Five**.

Fibre	The natural packaging of plant foods that are not digested in the small intestine. The chief categories are cellulose, hemicelluloses, pectins, gums, and lignins. Pectins and gums are viscous fluids rather than "fibrous". Some types of fibre increase the bulk of the feces and thereby relieve constipation and reduce **diverticula** formation in the colon. Pectin and guar gum slow gastric emptying and contribute to satiety.
	Dietary fibre is partly digested in the colon where it is fermented by gas-producing bacteria. The volatile fatty acids (acetic, butyric, or propionic) produced that contribute to colon health. "Soft" fibre, the kind best for humans, is found in vegetables, nuts, and fruits. "Hard" fibre is found in whole grain cereals and bran.
Free Radical	An oxidizing compound that is formed in the body or is induced by external agents (such as ultra violet rays, tobacco smoke and alcohol). Free radicals cause a lot of damage to cells and **DNA**. The body has means of neutralizing them by the use of **antioxidants**. The free radical is a molecule that contains at least one unpaired electron. Because of their odd electrons, free radicals are highly reactive. At worst they tear open intact molecules, cannibalizing parts of them to complete their own electron pairs and, in the process, generating new free radicals. Thus an exploding chain reaction is set in train that can cause huge damage out of all proportion to the initial provoking agent.
Fructose	A simple sugar (or monosaccharide) commonly found in fruit and in some vegetables. It sometimes combines with **glucose** to form a disaccharide, **sucrose** or table sugar. Fructose, unlike sugar, is slowly and harmlessly metabolized.
G.I.	See **Glycemic Index.**
Glucose	Also called dextrose, is a simple sugar (monosaccharide) found in fruits and honey. It is essential in just the right concentrations in the blood stream to supply energy to the muscles and the brain. Too high a level is known as **hyperglycemia**, too low a level is known as **hypoglycemia**.
Glycemic Index	This is a measure of what a carbohydrate does to blood sugar levels. The glycemic index (G.I.) for **glucose** (blood sugar) itself is defined as being 100. Most foodstuffs have an index less than 100. See Appendix One.
Granivore	A creature that gains most of its food supply from seeds. Granivores are chiefly birds. See **Chapter Four**.
Herbivore	Strictly speaking a herbivore is a creature that obtains most of its nutrition from grasses, like the cow, the horse and the sheep. Sometimes, but not in this book, a herbivore is defined as a creature that consumes mainly plant food. See **Chapter Four**.
Histamine	A chemical messenger involved in a number of complex biologic actions. It interacts with cell receptors to elicit changes in many different bodily functions. Histamine contracts muscles in the gut, the uterus, and the lungs; relaxes fine blood vessels; increases permeability of capillary walls; removes products of cell damage; combats allergens; stimulates stomach acid; stimulates the heart beat; modifies lymphocyte immune reactions. Histamine has a neurotransmitter role, but its function is unclear.
Hominoid	Creatures that have a human-like body shape. Technically any of a superfamily of primates including recent hominids, gibbons, and pongids together with extinct ancestral and related forms.
Hormone	Chemical messengers sent by one tissue in the body to instruct other tissues via the bloodstream. They regulate a host of bodily activities. Hormones are either steroids or amino acids (proteins).
Hydrogenated Oil and Trans-fatty Acids	These are much the same thing. They are made artificially by manufacturers who want to turn an oil solid at room temperature. In effect, they are converting polyunsaturated oils (like sunflower oil or corn oil) into **saturated fats**. They are commonly found in margarines and in many bakery products like cakes and cookies. These artificial fats are just as bad for health as real saturated fats. See **Chapter Five**.

Hyperglycemia	A state of abnormally high levels of glucose in the blood stream during which the excess glucose is directly toxic to the nervous system. See **Chapter Five**.
Hyperinsulinemia	A state of abnormally high levels of insulin in the bloodstream. See **Chapter Five**.
Hypoglycemia	A state of abnormally low levels of glucose in the bloodstream. Symptoms are varied but include mental impairment, irritability, sugar craving, confusion, tiredness, and seizures. See **Chapter Five**.
Insulin	**A** hormone secreted by the **pancreas** when blood sugar (glucose) rises. Its chief role is to encourage muscle and fat cells to take up glucose from the bloodstream and thereby reduce the blood sugar level down to normal. Insulin acts on many other body functions too. See **Chapter Five**.
Inulin	A sweet tasting substance that occurs particularly in roots and tubers such as the dahlia and the Jerusalem artichoke. The inulin molecule is a small, inert poly-saccharide that readily passes through the digestive system. Because the body does not absorb it, it has a low or zero G.I.
Irritable Bowel Syndrome	An extremely common disorder that is probably due to a disturbance of the motility of the whole intestinal tract. The symptoms vary from watery diarrhea to constipation and stomach cramps to nausea. See **Chapter Eight**.
Ischemic Heart Disease	An inadequate blood supply to a region of the heart due to a constriction or obstruction of a blood vessel.
Lactivore	A creature which obtains its nourishment from the milk of its mother. In practice this term applies to the unweaned young of mammals. See **Chapter Four**.
Law of Unintended Consequences	Fanciful term applied to the commonly observed phenomenon that people in trying to "fix" one problem often create unexpected side-effects that are worse than the original problem. See **Sorcerer's Apprentice Syndrome**.
Legume	Synonymous with **pulse.** Legumes are the dry fruit of the family Fabales. Important legumes are alfalfa, beans, broom, clover, lentil, pea, peanut, soybean and vetch. Legumes are high in protein.
Leukotriene	Any of a group of **eicosanoids** that participate in allergic responses. Leukotrienes are potent chemicals that dilate blood vessels and constrict bronchial air passages.
Micronutrient	A compound (as a vitamin, flavonoid or mineral) essential in minute amounts to growth and health.
Monounsaturated Fat	These are harmless **oils**, heat stable and most famously represented by olive oil. Although harmless, they are still empty calories and the body will be better off without them.
Oil	See **Fats and Oils.**
Omega 3 Oil	A family of **polyunsaturated oils** with the first double bond at the third position on the fatty acid chain. The **essential fatty acid** alpha-linolenic acid is the most important representative.
Omega 6 Oil	A family of **polyunsaturated oils** with the first double bond occurring at the sixth position on the fatty acid chain. The **essential fatty acid** linoleic acid is the most important representative.
Pancreas	The pancreas consists of two kinds of tissue: endocrine and exocrine. The latter produces pancreatic juice, a combination of digestive enzymes that empty via a duct into the small intestine.
	The endocrine tissues of the pancreas, the islets of Langerhans, secrete the hormones insulin and glucagon into the bloodstream.
pH	A measure of the acidity or alkalinity of watery solutions. pH ranges between 0 (most acidic) to 14 (most alkaline). Liquids that have a pH between 0 and 7 are acidic. Liquids that have a pH between 7 and 14 are alkaline. Pure water is neutral (neither acidic nor alkaline) and has a pH of 7. See **Chapter Five**.
Pleistocene	The Pleistocene Epoch began about 1,600,000 years ago and ended roughly 10,000 years ago. This was the time when our ancestors were evolving in tropical Africa in harmony with their environment.

Polyunsaturated Fat	A class of fat that has more than one double carbon bond. They are usually liquid at room temperature. There are two major families of polyunsaturated fats, **Omega 3** and **Omega 6**. They are chiefly represented by vegetable oils and marine (fish) oils.
Potassium	A soft, white, highly reactive metal with a silvery luster. In nature it is abundant in combination with other elements. In the human body it carries out, inter alia, essential cellular electrolytic functions in tandem with sodium. Potassium is found abundantly in vegetation, particularly some fruits. Chemical symbol, "K".
Primate	These are mammals that share many basic body characteristics and have been classified into the Primate Order. The Order comprises humans, apes, monkeys, and related creatures such as lemurs and tarsiers.
Prostaglandin	See **Eicosanoids.**
Protein	Complex molecules made up of **amino acids**. There are more than 50,000 different kinds of protein in the human body. They are the chief constituents of muscle, skin and blood cells and of **hormones**, **enzymes** and many other essential molecules.
	Proteins from animal sources like meat, fish, milk and poultry are sometimes known as "hard" proteins because they are harder to digest and metabolize. They contain problem constituents like sulfur and phosphorous that have to be disposed of by the liver.
	Plants contain proteins. **Legumes** and nuts (both of which are a form of seed) are particularly rich in protein, richer in many cases than animal protein. Young plants (like the ones that humans eat in salads and vegetables) are richer in protein than mature leaves. Proteins from plants are sometimes known as "soft" proteins since, on the whole, their digestion and metabolization are easier.
	Problems arise both when too much and too little protein is consumed. In general, people in the Western world eat far too much protein leading to diseases like acidosis, osteoporosis and kidney disease.
Pulse	The edible seeds of various leguminous crops (as peas, beans, or lentils). Used as a synonym for **legume**.
Purslane	A small, fleshy annual plant of the genus Portulaca, with prostrate, reddish stems, egg-shaped leaves attached by the narrower end, and small yellow flowers that open in the sunlight. From the earliest mentions by the ancient Greeks until recent times, purslane stems and leaves were eaten regularly as a salad or cooked like spinach. Today the variety "kitchen garden purslane" is still grown in Europe as a potherb.
	Purslane is remarkable for its richness in the **Omega 3** oil, alpha-linolenic acid, one of the success secrets of the Cretan diet (**Chapter Three**). Purslane is also extraordinarily rich in antioxidants such as alpha tocopherol, beta-carotene, vitamin C and glutathione. It is a great source of other micronutrients like calcium, phosphorous and iron. There is a movement to encourage the cultivation and consumption of this superbly nutritious vegetable.
Rickets	Also called vitamin D deficiency, is a disease of infancy and childhood characterized by defective bone growth and typified by bandy or bowed legs. In the absence of vitamin D, calcium is not properly absorbed and utilized by the body. Vitamin D is a steroid hormone that is produced in the skin by the action of sunlight. This is normally sufficient for most people and it is unnecessary to obtain vitamin D from food. People who live in high latitudes, or who do not often go out of doors, should nevertheless take pains to get some sunshine from time to time.
Saturated Fat	In a saturated fat, two hydrogen atoms are attached to each carbon atom (three on the terminal carbon atom). There are no carbon double bonds. In general, the more saturated fatty acids there are in a **triglyceride** the more solid it is at room temperature. Beef fat is highly saturated, chicken fat less so. The body has not been designed to work with most kinds of saturated fat. They block proper functioning of **essential fatty acids** and their **eicosanoids** resulting in diseases like heart disease, hardening of the arteries, thrombosis, high cholesterol levels and depressed immune system.

Savanna(h)	Any tropical or subtropical grassland characterized by scattered trees or shrubs, a dry season, and brush fires. African savanna grasses are either high grasses 5 to 15 feet tall or short grasses about 1 foot tall. The trees, many of which are acacia, are usually thorny and small-leafed. Groups of trees such as palms or cactus-like species and single trees such as baobabs are also common. There are large herds of grazing animals predated by lions, leopards and cheetahs. The bird life includes ostriches, eagles, falcons and vultures.
Sodium	A soft, malleable, highly reactive alkali metal with chemical symbol "Na". In compound form it is abundant in nature, especially as sodium chloride (table salt). It is needed by the body as a micronutrient for various biochemical reactions but salt in excess is harmful. Sodium occurs naturally in modest levels in most vegetation. This is about right for human requirements.
Sorcerer's Apprentice Syndrome	So-called after the Paul Dukas musical interpretation (l'Apprenti Sorcier) of Goethe's story made famous in Disney's Fantasia. In Fantasia Mickey Mouse, as the sorcerer's apprentice, has been given the task of fetching water from the well. To save himself the trouble, Mickey casts a spell on a broom to fetch the water for him. Unfortunately Mickey, who was meddling in matters he only half understood, didn't know the spell to *stop* the broom fetching water even though the tank was now full. The sorcerer's house filled up with water as the broom carried on inexorably fetching water as Mickey panicked.
	The Sorcerer's Apprentice Syndrome is the fanciful term applied to the commonly observed phenomenon that people in trying to "fix" one problem are often meddling in things they only half understand and thus make the situation worse. See **Law of Unintended Consequences**.
Starch	Consists of thousands of linked glucose units. Enzymes rapidly convert starch back to glucose. That is why starches have a high G.I. Starch is the main component of cereals, grains and potatoes.
Striation	A thin scratch mark as though made by a nail
Sucrose	A disaccharide consisting of conjoined glucose and fructose molecules. It is otherwise known as (table) sugar.
Sugars	Any of numerous sweet, colorless, water-soluble compounds present in the sap of seed plants and the milk of mammals. They make up the simplest group of carbohydrates. Sugars include **glucose** (dextrose); **fructose** (levulose); invert sugar, maltose; and lactose (milk sugar).
Thrombosis	The formation of a blood clot in the heart or in a blood vessel. Common causes are: injury to a blood vessel, "thick" blood (platelet stickiness), artery inflammation, fatty plaque formation (atherosclerosis), **aneurysm**, confinement in bed, abnormally large numbers of platelets, abnormally high levels of fats in the blood.
Thromboxane	Is any of a number of related hormones responsible for blood platelet agglomeration. Under the influence of thromboxanes, platelets adhere to one another and to blood vessel walls. Other prostaglandin mechanisms oppose platelet "stickiness" when necessary. Under many dietary errors explained in this book, this finely tuned mechanism is disrupted. On the whole, Westerners have a strong tendency to produce too much thromboxane and as a result suffer excessively from blood clotting disorders.
Trans-Fatty Acid	See **Hydrogenated Oil.**
Triglycerides	An ester of three fatty acids attached to a glycerol molecule. They are by far the most common form of fats in the diet and in the body. Triglycerides are deposited in animal tissues as storage for food energy. High triglycerides in blood circulation indicate either a high fat consumption or a poor metabolism of ingested fats. The body accumulates fat and metabolizes it as the energy requirements of the body demand it. See **Chapter Five**.
Vitamin F	Name given in the past in some countries to **essential fatty acids**. This use has not been formally adopted in scientific nomenclature but is still used informally, as in this work, as a useful shorthand for these vitamin-like substances.

Index

Principal references are in **bold**

THE BOND EFFECT RESOURCES

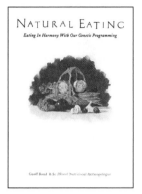

The Natural Eating
INTRODUCTORY GUIDE

The easy introduction to Natural Eating. In 32 pages it contains the distilled essence of the principles and practice. Produced in full colour and liberally illustrated with specially commissioned watercolours, it makes a superb gift for family, friends and colleagues.

The Natural Eating
MONTHLY NEWSLETTER

Densely packed pages of advertisement-free hints, tips and health up-dates on Natural Eating. It typically contains: Food/Disease Connections; Readers Questions and Answers; Practical Hints and Tips. Anthropological Notes; Quick-Fix Recipes; Food Label of the Month (Good or Bad); The Natural Eating view of Breaking News; Dining out (and in) strategies; Siren survival skills (marketing campaigns de-bunked); and much more.

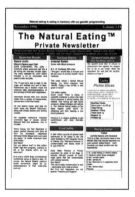

The Natural Eating
MANUAL

For the serious practitioner. It contains step-by-step implementation, precepts, charts, tables and detailed practical information. It is a hands-on practical specification for eating the Natural Eating way.

The Natural Eating
COOKBOOKS

The essential handmaidens to everyone living the Natural Eating Way. They contain interesting, tasty and practical recipes conforming to the Natural Eating precepts.

Speaking Engagements, breaking news, updates, hints and tips and much more.

Visit our web site
www.naturaleater.com

Enquiry Form

Yes please, send me without obligation, details of the following:

The Introductory Guide to Natural Eating ☐

The Natural Eating Newsletter ☐

The Natural Eating Manual ☐

The Natural Eating Cook Books ☐

Name	
Address 1	
Address 2	
City	
State/Country	
Postcode/Zip	
Telephone	
e-mail	

Post, fax or e-mail to:
Mail: Natural Eating, PMB 517, 69-115 Ramon Rd, #F1,
Cathedral City, CA 92234, USA.
fax: +1 (760) 328 8529, e-mail: info@naturaleater.com

✂